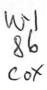
Advanced Practice in Healthcare

Advanced Practice in Healthcare outlines the key components of advanced practice in which healthcare professionals are engaged. With a clear skills focus, it explores issues critical to providing effective enhanced care to patients whilst managing and negotiating the complexities of the healthcare delivery system.

Perspectives on advanced practice are illuminated throughout the text and are designed to promote the formation of new thinking in relation to practice, education and research. The text is comprised of three sections that address different aspects of advanced practice and these in turn:

- Provide guidance on the development of clinical skills, including consultation, clinical decision making, holistic care, and the role of care planning in advanced practice;
- Explain management skills and how to manage, negotiate and monitor the complexities of the healthcare system in order to ensure the delivery of quality patient care;
- Clarify the professional role of the advanced practice clinician and how implementation of the role can improve the delivery of patient care.

In each chapter activities are presented that assist in the development, implementation and extension of advanced level practice. This text is especially relevant to nurses, midwives and allied health professionals practising within primary and secondary care who wish to advance their practice or clarify their roles within the context of advanced practice; particularly those undertaking masters level study.

Carol L. Cox is Professor of Nursing, Advanced Clinical Practice at City University London, UK.

Marie C. Hill is a Senior Lecturer in Practice Nursing at City University London, UK.

Victoria M. Lack is a Senior Urgent Care Practitioner at Harrogate District Hospital, North Yorkshire, UK.

'What has been missing for many is the opportunity to develop professional and managerial skills which will allow them to facilitate change and impact on health service policy and provision in their area of practice. This book addresses the professional skills and knowledge needed by these practitioners to ensure they can function effectively and efficiently in the variety of healthcare settings in which they practice, and consequently empower them to develop healthcare services which truly meet the needs of their service users. This text will be an essential resource for those already working in the advanced practice setting but will also inspire the nurse practitioners of the future. I certainly wish this text had been available to support me in my role development 20 years ago!'

Theresa Porrett, *PhD, MSc, Rn, Nurse Consultant in Coloproctology and Clinical Director, North East London Bowel Cancer Screening Centre, UK.*

'Cox, Hill and Lack have captured the essence of advanced practice within this book by providing a clear picture of what the role encompasses in today's complex health care systems. This book is useful not only for aspiring advanced practitioners, but also for established practitioners who wish to develop and enhance their practice even further. The contributors provide a comprehensive overview of the role which enables the reader to explore areas that impact upon this, both in the UK and Abroad. This book also offers a clear insight into a role that is wide ranging in that it includes key chapters on management, influencing others as well as clinical skills and decision making. Contributors from practice and academia share their expertise in a way in which the reader is engaged and allows them to question their own practice. I highly recommend this book.'

Anthony McGrath, *Department of Acute Health Care, University of Bedfordshire, UK.*

Advanced Practice in Healthcare

Skills for nurses and allied health professionals

Edited by
Carol L. Cox, Marie C. Hill and
Victoria M. Lack

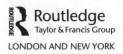
Routledge
Taylor & Francis Group

LONDON AND NEW YORK

First published 2012
by Routledge
2 Park Square, Milton Park, Abingdon, Oxon OX14 4RN

Simultaneously published in the USA and Canada
by Routledge
711 Third Avenue, New York, NY 10017

Routledge is an imprint of the Taylor & Francis Group, an informa business

British Library Cataloguing in Publication Data
A catalogue record for this book is available from the British Library

Library of Congress Cataloging-in-Publication Data
Advanced practice in healthcare: skills for nurses and allied health
professionals/edited by Carol Cox, Marie Hill, and Victoria Lack.
  p. ; cm.
  Includes bibliographical references.
  1. Nursing. 2. Allied health personnel. I. Cox, Carol Lynn.
  II. Hill, Marie C. (Marie Catherine), 1959–. III. Lack, Victoria.
  [DNLM: 1. Advanced Practice Nursing – methods. 2. Allied
  Health Personnel. WY 128]
  RT82.A38 2012
  610.73'7 – dc23   2011017868

ISBN: 978-0-415-59430-1 (hbk)
ISBN: 978-0-415-59431-8 (pbk)
ISBN: 978-0-203-35731-6 (ebk)

Typeset in Classical Garamond BT and Humanist 777 BT
by Florence Production Ltd, Stoodleigh, Devon

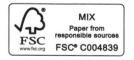

Printed and bound in Great Britain by
TJ International Ltd, Padstow, Cornwall

To Jim, Colin and Pete.
Thank you for all of your support.

Contents

Section II: Management

9   Influencing Others   **173**
Kathryn Waddington

Contributors

Rosa Benato
MSc, AMSPAR Dip Practice Management, PG Cert (Academic Practice), BSc (Hons)
Senior Lecturer, Education Development
Department of Public Health and Primary Care
School of Health Sciences
City University London

Elaine Cockram
PG Dip, BSc (Hons), RGN
Lead Nurse
Edgware Walk-in-Centre
Edgware, London

Carol L. Cox
PhD, MSc, MA Ed, PG Dip Ed, BSc (Hons), RN
Professor of Nursing, Advanced Clinical Practice
Department of Applied Biological Sciences
School of Health Sciences
City University London

Siobhan Hicks
PG Cert (Leadership), PG Cert (Academic Practice), BSc (Hons), NP Diploma Practice Nursing, RN
Lecturer in Advanced Clinical Practice
Department of Public Health and Primary Care
School of Health Sciences
City University London

Marie C. Hill
M.H.M., PG Dip, BSc (Hons), RN
Senior Lecturer, Practice Nursing
Department of Public Health and Primary Care
School of Health Sciences
City University London

Victoria M. Lack
MSc, PG Dip (Academic Practice), BN, DN Cert, RGN, FNP
Senior Urgent Care Practitioner
GP Out of Hours
Harrogate District Hospital
Harrogate, England

Jane Sumner
PhD, MN, BSN, Dip N, RN, APRN, BC
Professor of Nursing
Louisiana State University Health Sciences Center School of Nursing
New Orleans, LA, USA

Kathryn Waddington
PhD, MSc, PGCE (A), BSc (Hons), C Psychol, RN
Senior Lecturer, Director of Interprofessional Practice Programmes
Department of Interdisciplinary Studies in Professional Practice
School of Health Sciences
City University London

Ruth Walters
MSc, BA (Hons), RGN
Advanced Nurse Practitioner, Island Health Centre and
Clinical Lead, Healthy Island Partnership
London

Nicola Whiteing
MSc, PG Dip HE, BSc (Hons), RN, ANP
Senior Lecturer, Advanced Clinical Practice
Department of Applied Biological Sciences
School of Health Sciences
City University London

Foreword

Sir Jonathan Asbridge

The changing healthcare economy brings with it new challenges for healthcare professionals. Globally, healthcare organisations are experiencing radical revision to the way healthcare is provided and funded. Now, more than ever before, there is a need for all professional disciplines working within the healthcare sector throughout the world to assume aspects of advanced level practice. This may be in relation to their clinical skills provision, management abilities or as it relates to their leadership and professional roles.

To keep up with the pace of change in resources and technology we see a need for a blurring of boundaries in order to provide better, more holistic care to an expanding population. Blurring of boundaries implies assuming aspects of a variety of roles. There is an increasingly aging population that will require more complex and diversified services. With this comes a necessity for some healthcare professionals to become advanced level practitioners who will innovate and create new approaches to improve and maintain the health and wellbeing of our communities.

Advancing practice may be within the realm of clinical decision making, engaging in consultation, planning care, being an effective manager, negotiating and monitoring healthcare, behaving professionally, ensuring care is clinically effective or influencing others. All of these skills will need to be honed well to ensure front line clinical professionals can influence policy makers and funders to make the right strategic investment decisions and shape services which support advanced practitioners to deliver the most clinically effective and therefore cost-effective care. *Advanced Practice in Healthcare* is an insightful book that addresses the knowledge and skills advanced practitioners must master in order to lead these changes.

Sir Jonathan Asbridge, D. Sci., RGN
Programme Director – Healthy Futures Programme. North East Sector of Greater Manchester, England

Preface

This text has been written for the aspiring advanced level practitioner who wishes to launch their advanced level practice role as well as for the advanced level practitioner that wants to inform their thinking about changes and new developments associated with the healthcare professions. Throughout this book illuminating perspectives on practice emerge that will promote the formation of new thinking in relation to practice, education and research. In each chapter activities are presented to assist in the development, implementation and extension of advanced level practice.

In Section 1 of this text clinical skills are considered. Chapter 1 addresses consultation skills. Within the chapter, several models of consultation are presented. It then progresses to discuss methods of improving practice through the implementation of various aspects of these models. The chapter explores how consultation skills may be evaluated in practice. In Chapter 2, clinical decision making is examined. The chapter explores how clinical decisions can be made safely and effectively. It goes on to discuss how clinical governance, clinical evidence and research should influence the decision-making process. Chapter 3 delineates the role of care planning in advanced practice and explores specific skills that are needed to achieve holistic and realistic care planning in practice.

In Section 2 of this text management is considered. Chapter 4 reflects on management in terms of its definition and how management theory has evolved and developed. In addition, this chapter explores how management theories have influenced today's organisations and introduces activities that will help you develop and improve your management skills. Chapter 5 examines the role of the advanced practice nurse in healthcare delivery in the United States of America. It articulates the different specialties of advanced practice nursing and the various organisations that influence this role. Chapter 6 is designed to develop the knowledge, skills and strategies that promote effective management skills. There is a specific focus on the concept of emotional intelligence and how the principles of emotional intelligence can be applied to your own management practice.

Finally in Section 3 of this text, various aspects of leadership and the professional role are presented. There is an intention in this section to round out your development as well as extend your advanced level practice in relation to the key components of your leadership role. Chapter 7 describes the elements of professionalism associated with clinical/direct care advanced practice. In particular it considers professionalization as it relates to leadership and collaborative practice. Emphasis is placed on how you can improve the quality of care that is delivered and how you formulate plans for developing yourself and others at an advanced practice level. Chapter 8 provides you with background information about the importance of clinical effectiveness in relation to its three key elements. It discusses ways in which you can become involved in the implementation of evidence-based practice and develop your role as a case manager drawing on relevant domains and competencies of advanced level practice. Finally it provides guidance on tools to enable the collection of evaluative data on which to review practice. Chapter 9 is about influencing others in an organisation. The chapter draws upon theoretical perspectives and research from social and organisational psychology, public sector management and nursing, interwoven and applied to the emerging interdisciplinary field of interprofessional collaborative practice. When you have completed reading this chapter and engaging in its activities that are designed to enhance your learning you will be able to demonstrate an awareness of contemporary perspectives and theories of leadership and followership. You will have a sound understanding of various types of power and how you can use different influencing styles and tactics within a wider context of developing political awareness.

The authors that have contributed to this book are experts in the field of advanced practice. They have written each chapter with an intention of advancing and extending your practice. We think you will enjoy reading this text.

Carol L. Cox, Marie C. Hill and Victoria M. Lack

Introduction to Advanced Level Practice

Carol L. Cox,
Marie C. Hill and
Victoria M. Lack

Introduction

On 17 November 2010, the Department of Health published its position statement on advanced level practice. The position statement was developed in conjunction with the Department of Health's partners such as the Royal College of Nursing (RCN), UNISON, Skills for Health, the Nursing and Midwifery Council (NMC), NHS Employers, and the Department of Health Social Services and Public Safety. The position statement is intended to be used as a benchmark to enhance patient safety and the delivery of high quality care by supporting local governance, assisting in good employment practices and encouraging consistency in use of titles. Although the position statement has been developed primarily for nursing the Department of Health indicates that 'it may have relevance to midwifery, health visiting and allied health professions' (DoH, 2010:1). The Chief Nursing Officer for England, Dame Christine Beasley, indicated in the forward of the position statement that 'The health and social care landscape has changed dramatically over the years and new roles have emerged to respond to the complex and wide-ranging needs of people, families and communities' (DoH, 2010:2). Therefore it is evident that the changing healthcare system means the necessity for adapting on the part of healthcare professionals. Yet although the health professions have been and are adapting their practice, it can be presumed that they are remaining true to their core values (DoH, 2010). With this perspective in mind it is timely to clarify what advanced level practice is and its implications for further role development.

In this introductory chapter, advanced level practice will be addressed. A brief review of the background to advanced level practice will be presented firstly as it relates to the Council for Healthcare Regulatory Excellence (CHRE) published report in 2009, in which all healthcare professions were reviewed. The Department of Health position statement will be described and levels of practice defined. Subsequently the benchmark for advanced level practice will set the scene for reflecting on further development within the healthcare professions. Finally the context of advanced practice will be considered. Extensive quotes have been taken from the Department of Health (2010) position statement to ensure there is no misunderstanding about the Department of Health's position on advanced level practice.

Background

In 2008 the CHRE was asked by the Secretary of State for Health in the United Kingdom (UK) to examine advanced practice and to consider the necessity for regulation of advanced practice. The rationale for undertaking the review was to ensure that patient and public safety was not being put at risk because of advanced practice. The CHRE published its report in 2009 following its review. It found that there has been inconsistency in how the term 'advanced practice' has been applied to different healthcare professionals' roles. It indicated that this has frequently led to confusion about the scope and competence required at an advanced level of practice and confirmed the need for a set of nationally agreed standards for advanced level practice to support employers and commissioners in order to delineate good governance arrangements (CHRE, 2009; DoH, 2010).

The CHRE, in its 2009 UK-wide report, concluded that advanced practice was not a regulatory issue, and highlighted that:

- Risks to patient safety come from professionals taking on roles and responsibilities for which they are not competent to carry out safely and effectively, or because of inadequate safeguards;
- Employers are responsible for assessing fitness for purpose of their employees and job applicants with regard to the competencies (competence) required for the given job. Employers are in a position to determine this by considering the specific roles and responsibilities the professional would be taking on;
- Employers and commissioners need to ensure that robust organisational governance is in place to manage risks to patient safety from individuals in relation to competence and safeguards and that self-employed professionals are under a duty of care not to practise in ways in which they are not competent to do safely and to ensure that in the service they provide the necessary steps are taken to ensure patients are not put at unwarranted risk of harm and also that they keep their skills current in relation to their scope of practice;

- Core standards of the regulatory body emphasise the individual's role and responsibility as well as their accountability to the regulatory body when taking on activities for which they are capable of doing safely and effectively; generic standards should only be developed if a need is identified around a specific patient safety issue;
- Registered professionals must adhere to the duties specified by their regulatory body's core Code/Standards documents which make clear that they must only practise where they are capable of doing so safely and effectively, and should raise concerns and always act in the best interest of their patients if they feel they are being asked to work without appropriate safeguards. Self-employed professionals must ensure that they do not work without any safeguards necessary to protect the safety of their patients;
- Revalidation provides an opportunity for regulatory bodies to enhance governance of professional practice, by risk-assessing high risk activities and contexts and then identifying the evidence required for revalidation;
- Where professionals take on roles and responsibilities that are associated with another profession or a different regulatory body, it is important that professionals from both groups are regulated to appropriately similar standards;
- Professional bodies have a role in developing governance schemes to support the professional development of members and signal to employers the skill level a member has attained. They should issue additional guidance to members to assist them with ethical and practice issues which may arise which are benchmarked against the regulator's code. This is particularly where members are applying their knowledge and skills in new settings and contexts.

(CHRE:2009: Refer specifically to pp. 11–13)

In general, the CHRE report indicated that the primary issues associated with patient safety relate to practitioners not being competent and/or employers not providing safeguards. It concluded that a workforce that periodically demonstrates fitness for practice is more likely to be up-to-date and fit for purpose.

Interestingly, the Health Professions Council (HPC) took heed of the CHRE report acknowledging similarities within the allied health professions. The HPC supported the recommendations made by the CHRE regarding the regulation of advanced level practice. Although there was a view postulated by the CHRE that regulation of advanced practice was not necessary, it was clear that standards for advanced practice were required. 'It is the core role of the regulatory body to assure a professional's fitness to practise the profession, through setting and enforcing standards of proficiency and conduct' (CHRE, 2009:6).

The British government produced a statement in which it indicated that it supported the development of UK-wide standards for advanced practice in nursing, the allied health professions and for health care scientists. Midwifery was not mentioned in the statement as some midwives indicate that there is an advanced level of practice within the discipline whilst other midwives argue against this premise. The RCN indicates that advanced practice is a level of practice within the career framework of nursing (RCN, 2010a, 2010b). It is a level informed by the 'modernising nursing careers' work stream, of which the advanced practice component has been led by the Scottish Government Health Directorate. Competencies for advanced practice have been delineated and published by the RCN (2010a) and endorsed by the NMC. These were unveiled along with its position statement at the Nurse Practitioners Conference that was held in 2009 (RCN, 2010b).

The position statement published by the Department of Health responds to the need expressed by the CHRE in 2009 by defining the nature of advanced level nursing, what advanced practice encompasses and how advanced practice is different from the initial level of practice at registration. In the position statement the Department of Health indicates that 'it applies to all nurses involved in direct care delivery who work at an advanced level, regardless of area of practice, setting or client group. It describes a level of practice beyond that required to achieve registration. This statement seeks to improve understanding of advanced level practice and will help practitioners, commissioners, educators, service and workforce planners achieve their aim of building services focused on improving outcomes and experiences for patients' (Foreword by Dame Christine Beasley, DoH, 2010:2).

Advanced level practice position statement

The Department of Health (2010:3) position statement describes the level of practice expected of all 'nurses working at advanced level who provide direct care to patients, clients, service users or populations. It provides a benchmark for patients, carers, healthcare practitioners, managers, employers, commissioners and other stakeholders to use to make informed judgements regarding the required scope, level of practice and associated competence of nurses working at advanced level.' The statement has been informed by work that has been undertaken by organisations such as the Australian Nursing and

Midwifery Council (2009); Canadian Nurses Association (2008); Department of Health (2004); International Council of Nurses (2008); Nursing and Midwifery Council (2004); Royal College of Nursing (2010a); Scottish Government (2010) and Skills for Health (2006, 2009) to define and establish the competencies and standards for advanced practice in the UK and globally (DoH, 2010).

Levels of practice

Before defining what advanced level practice entails, it is important to review what is considered the preliminary level of practice (practice level on admission to the NMC register or to one of the HPC registers). For ease of consideration, nursing and the health professional will be addressed. The NMC (2008:1) indicates that all registered nurses are bound by The Code: Standards of Conduct, Performance and Ethics for Nurses and Midwives. This is also the norm for health professionals registered with the HPC (HPC, 2007). The HPC (2007:2) states: 'We expect you to keep to our Standards of Conduct, Performance and Ethics. Therefore it is evident that advanced level practice must be underpinned by a preliminary level of performance.' In relation to nursing, it can be seen that at the preliminary level:

- All registered nurses take personal responsibility for their actions and omissions, and fully recognise their personal accountability;
- All registered nurses are able to make sound decisions about their ongoing personal and professional development; practising within the scope of their personal professional competence and extending this scope as appropriate; delegating aspects of care to others and accepting responsibility and accountability for such delegation; and working harmoniously and effectively with colleagues, patients and clients and their carers, families and friends; and
- All registered nurses are expected to conduct themselves and practise within an ethical framework based upon respect for the well-being and safety of patients and clients.

(DoH, 2010:5)

The HPC (2007:2) maintains that standards of proficiency have been 'produced for the safe and effective practice of the professions we regulate. They are the minimum standards we consider necessary to protect members of the public'. In relation to health professionals, at the preliminary level:

The health professional must be able to:

- Recognise that they are personally responsible for and must be able to justify their decisions

1a.7   Recognise the need for effective self-management of workload and resources and be able to practise accordingly

1a.8   Understand the obligation to maintain fitness to practise

- Understand the need to practise safely and effectively within their scope of practice
- Understand the need to maintain high standards of personal conduct
- Understand the importance of maintaining their own health
- Understand both the need to keep skills and knowledge up to date and the importance of career-long learning

1b Professional relationships

Registrant physiotherapists must:

1b.1   Be able to work, where appropriate, in partnership with other professionals, support staff, service users and their relatives and carers

- Understand the need to build and sustain professional relationships as both an independent practitioner and collaboratively as a member of a team
- Understand the need to engage service users and carers in planning and evaluating diagnostics, treatments and interventions to meet their needs and goals
- Be able to make appropriate referrals
- Understand the structure and function of health, education and social care services in the UK and current developments, and be able to respond appropriately

1b.2   Be able to contribute effectively to work undertaken as part of a multi-disciplinary team

1b.3   Be able to demonstrate effective and appropriate skills in communicating information, advice, instruction and

Standards of proficiency 6 – Physiotherapists
Professional opinion to colleagues, service users, their relatives and carers:

- Be able to communicate in English to the standard equivalent to level 7 of the International English Language Testing System, with no element below 6.51
- Understand how communication skills affect the assessment of service users and how the means of communication should be modified to address and take account of factors such as age, physical ability and learning ability
- Be able to select, move between and use appropriate forms of verbal and non-verbal communication with service users and others
- Be aware of the characteristics and consequences of non-verbal communication and how this can be affected by culture, age, ethnicity, gender, religious beliefs and socio-economic status
- Understand the need to provide service users (or people acting on their behalf) with the information necessary to enable them to make informed decisions
- Understand the need to use an appropriate interpreter to assist service users whose first language is not English, wherever possible
- Recognise that relationships with service users should be based on mutual respect and trust, and be able to maintain high standards of care even in situations of personal incompatibility

1b.4   Understand the need for effective communication throughout the care of the service user

- Recognise the need to use interpersonal skills to encourage the active participation of service users

Standards of proficiency – Physiotherapists 7

1   'The International English Language Testing System (IELTS) tests competence in spoken and written English. Applicants who have qualified outside of the UK, whose first language is not English and who are not nationals of a country within the European Economic Area (EEA), have to provide evidence that they have reached the necessary standard. We accept a number of other tests as equivalent to the IELTS examination. Please visit our website for more information.'

(HPC, 2007:5–7)

Table I.1 clarifies the position of the Department of Health regarding advanced level practice in nursing in comparison to first level registration.

Advanced level nursing builds on and adds to the aforementioned statements expected of a nurse on admission to the NMC's register. The nurse working at an advanced level is expected to demonstrate expertise in all of the elements explicated by the Department of Health (2010). The definition of advanced level nursing focuses on the nature of advanced practice. It does not seek to classify types of roles as advanced practice roles or to specify pay structures. These components remain within the domain of employing organisations as specified by the CHRE in its 2009 report.

Benchmark for advanced level nursing

The benchmark for advanced level nursing provided in the position statement, according to the Department of Health, is generic. It 'applies to all clinical nurses working at an advanced level regardless of area of practice, setting or client group. It describes a level of practice, not specialty or role; that should be evident as being beyond that of first level registration. The benchmark should be viewed as a minimum threshold. It comprises 28 elements clustered under the following four themes (as agreed by expert practitioners):

- Clinical/direct care practice;
- Leadership and collaborative practice;
- Improving quality and developing practice; and
- Developing self and others.

(DoH, 2010:6)

TABLE I.1   Department of Health (2010) Perspective on Advanced Level Practice in Comparison to First Level Registration

Levels of Practice
The Department of Health recognises two levels of nursing practice: 'first level registration (entry into the profession) and advanced level, where the registered nurse is working at a level well beyond initial registration, using their existing knowledge and skills to inform and further develop their practice' (DoH, 2010:7). It should be noted that specific tasks do not define advanced level practice. 'What were once considered to be extended role activities – such as intravenous drug administration and cannulation – now form, following relevant preparation, the expected skills base of all registered nurses working in areas where these are key elements of nursing practice' (DoH, 2010:7).

All four themes and their associated elements must be demonstrable within the nurse's current role. All registered nurses should be continuously developing their practice and so it is anticipated that nurses working at advanced level will develop their practice beyond this threshold. The expectation is that nurses working at advanced level will have achieved this during extensive clinical/practice experience and following completion of Master's level education/learning or its equivalent (for example through Master's level postgraduate certificates/diplomas).

(DoH, 2010:6)

Definition of advanced level nursing practice

The Department of Health indicates that:

Advanced level practice encompasses aspects of education, research and management but is firmly grounded in direct care provision or clinical work with patients, families and populations. Nurses working at an advanced level promote public health and well-being. They understand the implications of the social, economic and political context of healthcare. Their expertise, experience and professional and clinical judgement are demonstrated in the expert nature of their practice and the depth of their knowledge. Patients, clients and other professionals acknowledge their highly developed and extensive knowledge in areas such as diagnostics, therapeutics, the biological, social and epidemiological sciences and pharmacology, and their enhanced skills in areas such as consultation and clinical decision making. Nurses working at an advanced level use complex reasoning, critical thinking, reflection and analysis to inform their assessments, clinical judgements and decisions. They are able to apply knowledge and skills to a broad range of clinically and professionally challenging and complex situations. Nurses working at advanced level act as practice leaders, they manage their own workload and work across professional, organisational, agency and system boundaries to improve services and develop practice. They network, locally, regionally and nationally. They assess and manage risk and proactively challenge others about risk.

Advanced level nursing involves constantly working to improve the quality of services and patient care. Advanced level nurses use a range of data, tools and techniques to improve practice and health outcomes and can demonstrate their impact and value. They develop productive relationships with numerous stakeholders in order to influence the strategic direction of services for the benefit of patients and clients.

Nurses working at advanced level are at the forefront of their area of practice.

They can identify their own and others' personal development needs and take effective action to address them. They are likely to have made best use of the wide range of learning and development opportunities available to them, learning not only through formal educational programmes but also from their own practice and from the individuals with whom they work. Such nurses will have a track record of innovative practice and service development, for example taking a lead in designing and delivering new care pathways and services and in the development and implementation of policy, standards, guidelines and protocols.

(DoH 2010:7–8)

Prior to the Department of Health undertaking its consultation on advanced level nursing, the NMC undertook a consultation on advanced practice nursing in 2004. It produced a consultation document on advanced practice for nurses in 2005 in which it indicated that these nurses:

- Take a comprehensive patient history;
- Carry out physical examinations;
- Use their expert knowledge and clinical judgement to identify the potential diagnosis;
- Refer patients for investigations where appropriate;
- Make a final diagnosis;
- Decide on and carry out treatment, including the prescribing of medicines, or refer patients to an appropriate specialist;
- Use their extensive practice experience to plan and provide skilled and competent care to meet patients' health and social care needs, involving other members of the health care team as appropriate;
- Ensure the provision of continuity of care including follow-up visits;
- Assess and evaluate, with patients, the effectiveness of the treatment and care provided and make changes as needed;
- Work independently, although often as part of a health care team; provide leadership; and
- Make sure that each patient's treatment and care is based on best practice.

(NMC, 2010:1)

As of February 2006 it was agreed that these were the definitive activities of the advanced nurse practitioner. In addition it indicated that 'Advanced nurse practitioners are highly experienced and educated members of the care team who are able to diagnose and treat your health care needs or refer you to an appropriate specialist if needed' (NMC, 2010:1). It is apparent when comparing the statements promulgated by the NMC in 2006 (NMC, 2010) and the Department of Health (2010) that there are significant similarities in the elements that comprise advanced level practice.

The Department of Health (2010) has specified elements of advanced level practice associated with the nationally agreed themes. The elements are shown in Table I.2 and can be viewed as being applicable to all healthcare professionals practising at an advanced practice level.

Advanced practice in context

Patricia Benner, in her seminal work 'from novice to expert' (1984), discusses the actions of expert nurses in their relations with doctors. She says that often expert nurses in intensive care know what the patient needs and have to find ways of communicating this to the doctors so that the right outcome is achieved. It is common knowledge that junior doctors often rely on the guidance and advice of experienced nurses to help them through their early career. However, even when nurses act in this expert role, it is the doctors who are ultimately responsible for the patient and who are responsible for the decisions made. Some nurses and other health care professionals in the past have chosen to take on the responsibility for the patient; for example in General Practice where practice nurses have routinely managed chronic disease clinics, initiated and altered treatment regimes and filled in blank prescriptions for many years. However, even here, although the nurse may want to have the responsibility, it is ultimately the general practitioner GP who remains responsible for the patient. The GP was, until recently, the individual signing the prescription. This is where expert practice differs from advanced practice. Advanced practitioners are autonomous practitioners and make their own decisions, follow them through and are responsible for all of the care provided. Many nurses will know what the right course of action is for a patient, but it is not their role to make the final decision in relation to healthcare provision. Advanced practitioners must be prepared to make the final decision and live with the consequences. In order to be able to do this, advanced practitioners must have the knowledge required to make the decisions and be prepared to take risks. They must have the intelligence to solve complex problems and the professional integrity to lead and develop their profession. This role is not one that many health professionals will

TABLE 1.2 Themes and Elements of Advanced Level Practice

Nationally Agreed Themes and Elements of Advanced Level Practice

1 Clinical/direct care practice

Healthcare practitioners working at an advanced level:

1.1 practise autonomously and are self-directed;
1.2 assess individuals, families and populations holistically using a range of different assessment methods, some of which may not be usually exercised by them such as physical/clinical examination, ordering and interpreting diagnostic tests or advanced health needs assessment;
1.3 have a health promotion and prevention orientation, and comprehensively assess patients for risk factors and early signs of illness;
1.4 draw on a diverse range of knowledge in their decision-making to determine evidence-based therapeutic interventions (which will usually include prescribing medication/treatments and actively monitoring the effectiveness of therapeutic interventions);
1.5 plan and manage complete episodes of care, working in partnership with others, and delegating and referring as appropriate to optimise health outcomes and resource use, as well as providing direct support to patients and clients;
1.6 use their professional judgement in managing complex and unpredictable care events and capture the learning from these experiences to improve patient care and service delivery;
1.7 draw upon an appropriate range of multi-agency and inter-professional resources in their practice; and
1.8 appropriately define the boundaries of their practice.

2 Leadership and collaborative practice

Healthcare practitioners working at an advanced level:

2.1 identify and implement systems to promote their contribution and demonstrate the impact of advanced level practice to the healthcare team and the wider health and social care sector;
2.2 provide consultancy services to their own and other professions on therapeutic interventions, practice and service development;
2.3 are resilient and determined and demonstrate leadership in contexts that are unfamiliar, complex and unpredictable;
2.4 engage stakeholders and use high-level negotiating and influencing skills to develop and improve practice;
2.5 work across professional, organisational and system boundaries and proactively develop and sustain new partnerships and networks to influence and improve health, outcomes and healthcare delivery systems;
2.6 develop practices and roles that are appropriate to patient and service need through understanding the implications of and applying epidemiological, demographic, social, political and professional trends and developments; and
2.7 identify the need for change, proactively generate practice innovations and lead new practice and service redesign solutions to better meet the needs of patients and the service.

continued ...

TABLE 1.2   Themes and Elements of Advanced Level Practice ... *continued*

3 Improving quality and developing practice

Healthcare practitioners working at an advanced level:

3.1   are proactively involved in developing strategies and undertaking activities that monitor and improve the quality of healthcare and the effectiveness of their own and others' practice;

3.2   strive constantly to improve practice and health outcomes so that they are consistent with or better than national and international standards through initiating, facilitating and leading change at individual, team, organisational and system levels;

3.3   continually evaluate and audit the practice of self and others at individual and systems levels, selecting and applying valid and reliable approaches and methods which are appropriate to needs and context, and acting on the findings;

3.4   continually assess and monitor risk in their own and others' practice and challenge others about wider risk factors;

3.5   critically appraise and synthesise the outcomes of relevant research, evaluations and audits and apply the information when seeking to improve practice;

3.6   plan and seize opportunities to generate and apply new knowledge to their own and others' practice in structured ways which are capable of evaluation;

3.7   alert appropriate individuals and organisations to gaps in evidence and/or practice knowledge and, as either a principal investigator or in collaboration with others, support and conduct research that is likely to enhance practice; and

3.8   use financial acumen in patient/client, team, organisational and system level decision-making and demonstrate appropriate strategies to enhance quality, productivity and value.

4 Developing self and others

Healthcare practitioners working at an advanced level:

4.1   actively seek and participate in peer review of their own practice;

4.2   enable patients/clients to learn by designing and coordinating the implementation of plans appropriate to their preferred approach to learning, motivation and developmental stage;

4.3   develop robust governance systems by contributing to the development and implementation of evidence-based protocols, documentation processes, standards, policies and clinical guidelines through interpreting and synthesising information from a variety of sources and promoting their use in practice;

4.4   work in collaboration with others to plan and deliver interventions to meet the learning and development needs of their own and other professions;

4.5   advocate and contribute to the development of an organisational culture that supports continuous learning and development, evidence-based practice and succession planning; and

4.6   have high-level communication skills and contribute to the wider development of those working in their area of practice by publicising and disseminating their work through presentations at conferences and articles in the professional press.

(DoH, 2010:9–11)

aspire to or want. However, for those that do and who achieve the role of an advanced practitioner, the professional reward is worth the effort and risk involved.

The advanced level role has however suffered from a lack of clarity and recognition in the UK. The nurse practitioner in the United States is recognised by public and professionals alike, as an individual that is a competent professional with postgraduate training and passed a national examination enabling them to practice independently. Along with this comes the right to prescribe, make referrals and initiate investigations and also to charge for these services. In the UK there is not such understanding or recognition. The CHRE (2009) report lays the burden of competence firmly with the employer to enforce. To date employers have not done this. Conversely employers have added to the confusion by introducing a plethora of titles for nurses with very varying skills. This is the reason why there is so much misunderstanding among health professionals, not to mention the general public, about what exactly a nurse practitioner (or advanced practitioner) is or can do. Coupled with this, there are examples of advanced practice around the country that have not been well documented, evaluated or made sustainable. In the words of the reviewers of advanced practice roles for skills for health:

> Advanced practitioner roles have had distinct benefit [for patients], which for various reasons, trusts have found difficult to document. The need to improve the evidence base on Advanced Practice role impact gives rise to two main challenges: securing resources to implement the roles to ensure they are sustainable, and how best to diffuse innovation across the NHS.
>
> (Miller, Cox and Williams, 2009:viii)

The report goes onto say that like many 'good ideas' advanced practice roles are not being systematically spread across the NHS trusts or regions. We seem to be caught in a perpetual pilot project stage. A slightly cynical reason for this is that employers are quite happy to let the status quo continue where nurses are 'acting up' without sufficient recognition and perhaps training as this appears initially to be the more cost effective option. This unfortunately invites unconscious incompetence all round. It is reassuring that the Department of Health (2010) recognises the distinct role of advanced practitioners and the education required to fulfil this role. What is still unclear is how the advanced practice level role will be made distinct and apparent to professionals and the public. It is also unclear how advanced practice education will be financed and regulated in order to achieve and maintain the necessary standards for the protection of advanced practitioners and the public alike.

It is important, however, to be positive about how far advanced practice has come in the UK in the last 20 years. There are many advanced practitioners in dynamic roles that are continuously developing practice to the advantage of individuals and communities. Many of these practitioners have some prescribing and referral rights, which facilitate holistic care. It is good to be able to make the final decision and not rely on the decisions of others who may not share the same opinion. It is good to have to justify your own prescribing habits and not rely on the prescribing habits of others. It is good to have the knowledge or have access to the knowledge to make rational decisions. It is good to be able to care for patients holistically because you have the capacity to do so.

It is good that advanced practice is now being recognised as a distinct entity requiring years of preparation at post-graduate level. This is great progress. We need to continue to develop this new professional group of advanced practitioners into a cohesive recognisable entity, albeit with differing backgrounds and areas of expertise. It must be hoped that patients and communities will benefit from our skills and also that a new and dynamic group of people will be attracted to join the ranks of advanced level practitioners.

Conclusion

This chapter has introduced the aspiring and established advanced level practice nurse, midwife or allied health professional to the most recent perspectives regarding advanced practice. It has described the concept of advanced level practice from the perspective of the Council for Healthcare Regulatory Excellence (2009), the Department of Health (2010), the Health Professions Council (2007), the Nursing and Midwifery Council (2010), Royal College of Nursing (2010a) and other associated healthcare organisations. It has delineated elements, domains and competencies that are integral to the role of advanced level practice. The chapter has considered issues associated with regulation of advanced level practice and indicated that it is hoped that patients, carers, their families and the health service benefit from the implementation of advanced practice roles.

In the chapters that follow, various concepts associated with clinical skills, management, leadership and the professional role in advanced level practice are explicated. Specific activities are embedded in the chapters. These activities are designed for your personal reflection and development.

References

Australian Nursing and Midwifery Council (2009) *Nurse Practitioners: Standards and Criteria for the Accreditation of Nursing and Midwifery Courses Leading to Registration, Enrolment, Endorsement and Authorisation in Australia – with Evidence Guide*. Available from: http://www.anmc.org.au/userfiles/file/ANMC_Nurse_Practitioner(1).pdf (accessed 14/06/2011)

Benner, P. (1984) *From novice to expert: Excellence and power in clinical nursing practice*. Menlo Park, California: Addison-Wesley.

Canadian Nurses Association (2008) *Advanced Nursing Practice: A National Framework*. Available from: http://www.cna-aiic.ca/CNA/documents/pdf/publications/ANP_National_Framework_e.pdf (accessed 14/06/2011)

Council for Healthcare Regulatory Excellence (2009) *Advanced Practice: Report to the Four UK Health Departments. Unique ID 17-2008*. Available from: http://www.chre.org.uk/_img/pics/library/090709_Advanced_Practice_report_FINAL.pdf (accessed 14/06/2011)

Department of Health (2004) *The NHS Knowledge and Skills Framework (NHS KSF) and the Development Review Process*. Available from: http://www.dh.gov.uk/en/Publicationsandstatistics/Publications/PublicationsPolicyAndGuidance/DH_4090843 (accessed 14/06/2011)

—— (2010) *Advanced Level Nursing: A Position Statement*. http://www.dh.gov.uk/prod_consum_dh/groups/dh_digitalassets/@dh/@en/@ps/documents/digitalasset/dh_121738.pdf (accessed 14/06/2011)

Health Professions Council (2007) *Standards of Proficiency: Generic Statement*. Available from: http://www.hpc-uk.org/aboutregistration/standards/standardsofproficiency/index.asp (accessed 14/06/2011)

International Council of Nurses (2008) *The Scope of Practice, Standards and Competencies of the Advanced Practice Nurse*. International Council of Nurses, Geneva.

Miller L., Cox A. and Williams J. (2009) *Report 465: Evaluation of the advanced practitioner roles:* Brighton: Institute for Employment Studies.

Nursing and Midwifery Council (2004) *Consultation on a Framework for the Standard for Post-registration Nursing*. Available from: http://www.nmc-uk.org/Documents/Consultations/NMC%20Consultation%20-%20port%20registration%20nursing%20-%20consultation%20document.pdf (accessed 14/06/2011)

—— (2005) *Implementation of a Framework for the Standard for Post Registration Nursing. Agendum 27.1 December 2005/c/05/160* Available from: http://www.nmc-uk.org/Get-involved/Consultations/Past-consultations/By-year/The-proposed-framework-for-the-standard-for-post-registration-nursing--February-2005/ (accessed 14/06/2011)

—— (2008) *The Code: Standards of Conduct, Performance and Ethics for Nurses and Midwives*. Available from: http://www.nmc-uk.org/Nurses-and-midwives/The-code/The-code-in-full/ (accessed 14/06/2011)

—— (2010) Available from: http://www.nmc-uk.org/Get-involved/Consultations/Past-consultations/By-year/The-proposed-framework-for-the-standard-for-post-registration-nursing – February-2005/ (accessed 14/06/2011)

Royal College of Nursing (2010a) *Advanced Nurse Practitioners – An RCN Guide to the Advanced Nurse Practitioner Role, Competences and Programme Accreditation*. Available from: http://www.rcn.org.uk/__data/assets/pdf_file/0003/146478/003207.pdf (accessed 14/06/2011)

—— (2010b) Available from: http://www.rcn.org.uk/newsevents/congress/2010/congress_2010_resolutions_and_matters_for_discussion/20._advance_regulation_for_advanced_nursing (accessed 14/06/2011)

Scottish Government (2010) *Advanced Nursing Practice Roles: Guidance for NHS Boards*. Available from: http://www.advancedpractice.scot.nhs.uk/media/19742/microsoft%20word

%20-%20sg%20advanced%20practice%20guidance%20-%20final%20mar%2010.pdf (accessed 14/06/2011)

Skills for Health (2006) *Career Framework*. Available from: http://www.skillsforhealth.org.uk/developing-your-organisations-talent/more-efficient-workforce-planning/public-health-career-framework/ (accessed 14/06/2011)

—— (2009) *Nationally Transferable Roles.* http://www.skillsforhealth.org.uk/rethinking-roles-and-services/proven-role-templates-for-a-skilled-and-flexible/ (accessed 14/06/2011)

Section I **Clinical Skills**

Chapter 1   **Clinical Decision Making**

*Elaine Cockram and
Siobhan Hicks*

Introduction

Clinical decision making is an integral part of clinical practice. One of the vital functions of an Advanced Practitioner (AP) is to be able to differentiate between patients that need more urgent treatment and assessment from those that don't. Clinical decision making is a learned skill, which is developed alongside increasing knowledge and experience. It appears different clinicians use various methods to make decisions, albeit mostly unconsciously, and the same clinician may use different methods depending on the complexity of the situation and the familiarity of the clinician with it. What does seem to be apparent is that practitioners require a substantial knowledge of the subject area before safe and effective decisions can be made. It is therefore necessary to have access to resources to facilitate decision making as not all knowledge necessary can be retained. Clinical decision making is not only about the individual clinician and their skills, it is also about the ability of the organisation as a whole to ensure clinical decisions are made with the most up to date evidence available so that quality and equality are attained. This concept, embedded in clinical governance, will be examined in the second half of the chapter. Finally clinical support is also needed from colleagues and the organisation in order to achieve and maintain safe decision making skills.

Learning outcomes

At the conclusion of this chapter you will be able to:

*   Discuss the steps involved in clinical decision making
*   Explore what knowledge is necessary in order to make effective clinical decisions
*   Understand the importance of clinical governance in terms of client safety and professional development
*   Discuss the benefits of clinical supervision within the clinical governance agenda.

Background

In order to engage in appropriate clinical decision making, Advanced Practitioners (APs) need to have subject-specific knowledge as a prerequisite (Botti and Reeve, 2003). Haynes et al. (2002) agree with this, saying that clinical expertise involves knowledge of the patient's clinical condition, knowledge of research-based evidence and patient preferences. Thompson and Dowding (2002), in what they call 'evidence-based decision making', say this involves combining clinical expertise, patient preferences and research evidence. Therefore, clinical decision making involves research based knowledge, physical assessment skills and communication. However, clinical decision making does not just require knowledge. It requires the application of that knowledge in order to formulate a diagnosis and plan of action in areas where nurses and other healthcare professionals (HCPs) would traditionally defer to a medical colleague. According to Bloom's Taxonomy (Bloom, 1956), diagnosis is an analytical skill involving critical thinking. This is reflected in the Nursing and Midwifery Council's (NMC) advice regarding training of Advanced Nurse Practitioners (ANPs) in that it should involve 'M level thinking' (NMC, 2005a). Most nurses in England have traditionally been educated at diploma level, where critical thinking is usually not required and is not assessed. The question therefore is: How can and do nurses move from a level of thinking that involves knowledge and comprehension, onto a level where they are able to apply knowledge and begin to analyse that knowledge? For example, where they are using the skill of critical thinking? This may be an important issue for nurses but is less so for other non-medical clinicians, as training is usually at degree level. At degree level many non-medical clinicians are taught decision making models and how to think critically.

Bloom's (1956) theoretical model analysis shows the cognitive functions involved in decision making. The functions are classified into six dynamic levels of increasing complexity as shown below in Table 1.1.

There is ordinarily a sequential progression from knowledge to comprehension, to application, to analysis, to synthesis and finally evaluation. Therefore, in order to be able to make a competent clinical diagnosis the clinician must be able to:

- Obtain and appreciate the meaning of symptoms and signs of the patient
- Identify the appropriate organ system/s involved in disease
- Speculatively identify the possible pathological processes that is/are occurring

- Know how to differentiate one pathological process from the other
- Know from epidemiology the most likely causes of particular pathological processes
- Evaluate all pieces of information available and decide on the likely cause and course of illness.

TABLE 1.1 Cognitive functions involved in clinical decision making

Cognitive level	Keywords	Usage in case presented
1. Knowledge	Recognition, recall	Recognition of symptoms and signs
2. Comprehension	Translation	Assigning signs and symptoms to systems, i.e. vomiting and diarrhoea to gastrointestinal
3. Application	Relate, transfer associate	Relating signs and symptoms to pathological conditions, i.e. diarrhoea to gastro-enteritis or colitis
4. Analysis	Distinguish, discriminate	Picking out the specific (which are key disease indicators) from the non-specific
5. Synthesis	Formulate, combine	Putting features together into a recognisable pattern for a specific condition or conditions
6. Evaluation	Validate, argue, reconsider, appraise	Checking if the diagnosis explains all signs and symptoms, identifying any symptoms that are not easily explained and the features of the diagnosed condition that are missing

Adapted from Bloom, 1956.

The decision making process

There has been a lot of interest dating from the seminal work by Patricia Benner in the late 1980's (Benner and Tanner, 1987) surrounding the issue of how nurses make decisions. Patricia Benner advocates that nurses tend towards a humanistic-intuitive approach to decision making, whereas a more systematic approach is put forward by Bench-Capon (1990) and others. However, these approaches described are based around work with general nurses; advanced nurse practitioners may use other methods, and indeed may need to use other methods in their work. In studies examining how health professionals in general make clinical decisions, two main models emerge: In the hypothetico-deductive method, the clinician derives hypotheses from the patient's presenting complaint that drives data collection and decision making (Offredy, 1998). In the pattern-matching model, clinicians use key clues to identify patterns that they recognise, and make their decisions according to their previous experience with that pattern of symptoms and signs (Mandin et al.,1997). Benner's (1987) concept of intuition has been examined separately, and may seem to be linked to the pattern-matching method, although with intuition, the process of decision making happens subconsciously (Offredy, 1998).

Obviously, both with pattern-matching and intuition, this relies on a significant level of experience. Therefore, it would seem that novices will make decisions in a different way from experienced practitioners (Burman et al., 2002). This is seen also with newly qualified and experienced nurse practitioners (Offredy, 1998). However, Offredy notes that experienced nurse practitioners will return to the hypothetic-deductive model when faced with an unknown situation. What is most interesting is that the methodology of clinical decision making matters less than mastery of the domain (Offredy, 1998). An article in the British Medical Journal (BMJ) from 2002, by Elstein and Schwarz, reviewed the literature surrounding the issues of clinical problem solving and diagnostic decision making by doctors. They also found, in the review, that accuracy in diagnosis depends less on the strategy used as on mastery of the content and suggest that experienced medical practitioners are effective at diagnosing problems because they use pattern recognition or retrieval of knowledge. They will use a deductive strategy only in difficult cases, as was found to be the case with nurse practitioners. They say the educational implication of this is that problem-based learning (the case study approach) is beneficial to students as it can teach the testing of clinical hypotheses to students, before they encounter real patients. Since almost any care will be complex for students, teachers should facilitate the hypothesis testing approach. Clinicians will then use the pattern-recognition approach as they become more experienced.

Activity 1

Think of a consultation where you were able to reach a diagnosis by pattern-matching and one where you had to use a deductive approach. What resources did you need in order to achieve a diagnosis in the second case?

Clinical reasoning techniques

Skills in clinical decision making can be consciously developed by thinking critically during history taking. For example, you can challenge yourself by asking yourself WHY and WHAT IF and then mapping diagnostic possibilities. It might be easier at first to write everything down in a mind map. You can then explore different hypotheses, where the diagnostic possibilities written down are upgraded depending on the presenting symptoms and signs. For example, somebody attending with ear pain could be upgraded from otitis externa to mastoiditis if they also have fever, feel unwell and have pain and inflammation over the mastoid area. You could also do this by thinking of red flags first and then working downwards. In practice the question 'What is the worst thing this could be?' should be the first question for less experienced APs in order to achieve safe practice.

Patient shared decision making

In shared decision making the intention is that through a collaborative process of decision making, the treatment decision will be shared between clinician and patient. When choosing a treatment or preventive procedure the aim is for us to select options that increase the likelihood of desired health outcomes and minimise the chance of undesired consequences. These undesired consequences may be detected with our conscious processing and as we come across information which fails to fit acceptable patterns. When deciding on a differential diagnosis clinicians may have a good idea about the probable cause but sometimes it is perfectly reasonable to wait and see. For example a young child presenting with otitis media will be in pain which is distressing for the parent. A good explanation of the aetiology of the illness and the necessity of adequate analgesia rather than antibiotics will usually pacify the parent. Giving them the information that they require and the option to obtain antibiotics if the pain is not subsiding is a good example of shared decision making. Ideally this incorporate. the patient's preferences as well as research evidence and knowledge of the patient's clinical state.

Emotional intelligence

We rely on our emotions and how we can control them. Emotions are functional and adaptive; they organize our thinking and motivate our behaviour and help us know what to pay attention to. Daniel Goleman (1998) indicates that emotional competence is a learned capability based on emotional intelligence that then results in outstanding performance at work. People with a high level of emotional intelligence will probably be more likely to be confident and competent with their clinical decision making. This is because they will be more likely to be empowered to learn the required skills to develop the ability and confidence to make important decisions.

Goleman (1998) proposes a framework of personal competencies that stem from the emotional intelligence concept. Typically, to achieve outstanding performance several of these skills are required. These are spread out among five domains which are self-awareness, self-regulation, motivation, empathy and social skills.

By the very nature of their work, clinicians are often faced with profound, moving, and sometimes disturbing experiences. These experiences have the potential to catalyze personal growth. Clinicians achieve a great deal of satisfaction when they know that they have managed such a case competently. Encouraging 'success' enhances problem-solving capabilities through the promotion of positive notions of self-concept and self-efficacy (Berger, 1984).

TABLE 1.2 Emotional Intelligence

Self-awareness Knowing one's internal states, preferences, resources and intuitions	Emotional awareness: *Recognizing one's emotions and their effects* Accurate self-assessment: *Knowing one's strengths and limits* Self-confidence: *A strong sense of one's self-worth and capabilities*
Self-regulation Managing one's internal impulses and resources	Self-Control: *Keeping disruptive emotions and impulses in check* Trustworthiness: *Maintaining standards of honesty and integrity* Conscientiousness: *Taking the responsibility for personal performance* Adaptability: *Flexibility in handling change* Innovation: *Being comfortable with novel ideas, approaches, and new information*
Motivation Emotional tendencies that guide or facilitate reaching goals	Achievement drive: *Striving to improve or meet a standard of excellence* Commitment: *Aligning with goals of the group or organization* Initiative: *Readiness to act on opportunities*
Personal Skills How we manage ourselves	Optimism: *Persistence in pursuing goals despite obstacles and setbacks*
Social skills	Communicating and relating to others: *Listening openly and sending convincing messages*

(Goleman, 1998)

In order to effectively make clinical decisions the clinician must perceive that they actually can make the decision; particularly when the situation is more challenging. Like so many things in life, in order to become proficient in any physical or mental process, it is necessary to be motivated. Decision making is enhanced when you listen and learn; then incorporate what you already know, blend it altogether and then often a decision will emerge.

Biases and preconceptions

Be aware of the number of biases that may lead you to poor decision making, i.e., subjective and objective impressions of the patient may lead to faulty assumptions regarding the patient's abilities or illnesses. For example, a patient who appears frail and thin may be viewed as being seriously ill or unable to participate in activities of daily living when in fact they may not be incapacitated in any way. To counter faulty assumptions, biases, and preconceptions, it is important to ensure that you continually validate information and your impressions through the use of data gathering and effective interviewing techniques.

Clinical governance

In considering the notion of risk for the advanced practitioner, it is undeniable that lifelong education, experience and organisational support are central factors in reducing harm when making decisions in clinical practice. Clinical governance aims to put quality at the heart of health care, in order to sustain and improve high standards. It is 'the process by which each part of the National Health Service (NHS) quality assures its clinical decisions by introducing a system of continuous improvement into the operation of the whole NHS.' (DoH, 1998:33).

Domain 6 of the Royal College of Nursing (RCN, 2010) Competencies for Advanced Practice: Monitoring and Ensuring the Quality of Advanced Health Care Practice, states that ANPs should monitor the quality of their own practice and participate in continuous quality improvement and evaluate patient follow up and outcomes including consultation and referral. One activity that can be beneficial in assuring that this competency is met is to keep a record of consultations. This can then be used to facilitate the review and follow up of the client's attendance, re-attendance, treatment, diagnosis, referral and follow up. The format chosen for recording is flexible and may include writing a daily diary entry/blog or by using a spreadsheet (refer to example 1 below). This ongoing exercise builds a written memory of knowledge and experience, facilitating reflection on personal and professional development as an ANP. In the words of Franklin P. Jones (unknown), 'Experience is that marvellous thing that enables you to recognize a mistake when you make it again.'

Example 1

Date	ID	Age	Complaint	Diagnosis	Treatment	Referral	Follow up	Notes
		19	Abdominal pain	? Appendicitis	Refer	Surgical team	Admitted	Appendectomy
		3	Ear pain	Viral URTI	OTC analgesia	Pharmacy	Did not reattend	
		75	Discharge from wound	Infected laparotomy wound site	Oral flucloxacilin	None	Did not reattend	
		8	Sore throat	Viral tonsillitis	OTC analgesia	Pharmacy	Reconsulted General Practitioner 2 days later	Given oral penicillin v.

Activity 2

How can you audit your clinical decision making skills in practice?

An educated, trained and developed workforce is an integral part of clinical governance. There is considerable support available now for advanced practitioners in practicing evidence based medicine: NHS clinical guidelines are available from the National Institute for Health and Clinical Excellence (NICE, 2011) http://www.nice.org.uk/, The Scottish Intercollegiate Guidelines Network (SIGN) http://www.sign.ac.uk/ and Clinical Knowledge Summaries http://www.cks.nhs.uk/home. Modular learning is available from the BMJ http://learning.bmj.com/learning/main.html and charities such as Diabetes United Kingdom (UK) http://www.diabetes.org.uk/ and the National Eczema Society http://www.eczema.org/. All of these organisations have online resources for professionals. There is support for educators from the Association of Advanced Nurse Practitioner Educators (AANPE) who liaise closely with the RCN, the RCN Nurse Practitioner Association and the NMC in order to represent a collaborative network of Higher Education Institutions across the

United Kingdom providing advanced clinical programmes of education for nurses. Additionally, employers may access tools to look at new ways of working, The Skills for Health (2010) website http://www.skillsforhealth.org.uk/ provides information and suggestions for developing competencies, frameworks and learning and development needs for advanced practice roles. These have been mapped against the Knowledge and Skills Framework (KSF, 2005; NHS, 2005b) which embraces the principles of clinical governance by encouraging training, assessment of competence, on-going supervision and risk management. Most of these resources are available free at the point of use and are accessible to all clinicians. It is the aim of clinical governance to provide a comprehensive range of guidelines to facilitate evidenced based practice and to a large extent this is being achieved. There is little excuse to say that the knowledge is unavailable to assist in clinical decision making.

The competencies for Advanced Practice, from the RCN (2010) and the Nursing and Midwifery Council (NMC, 2005a), largely agree standards for advanced level practice which facilitate the regulation of advanced practice at a local level. Recent findings by the Council for Healthcare Regulatory Excellence (CHRE, 2009) support this; but there is still concern about the recognition of the title for advanced practice nurses. The CHRE report states that much of what is often called advanced practice appears to represent career development and not a fundamental break with a profession's practice, such that the risks to the patient safety are adequately captured by the existing standards of proficiency, making additional statutory regulation largely unnecessary. Therefore the report does not see that additional regulation and a separate register or part of the register for ANPs is necessary. However, ANPs and other advanced practitioners, make complex clinical decisions, diagnose and prescribe treatment. In effect they are moving beyond nursing practice or other allied healthcare practice to incorporate elements of medical practice into their role. This demands much higher autonomy and accountability in practice. With this in mind it may be prudent to remember the Bolam Test (CHRE, 2009), which reminds us about the duty of care to our patients; that if we are negligent we will be judged against the standard of the ordinary skilled man who exercises that skill or profession. In the case of APs this would be another AP or a doctor.

An example of organisational governance that can aid APs in general practice is the Quality Outcomes Framework (QOF) (DoH, 2003) which monitors clinical practice and audits significant events in order to reflect upon, reduce the risk of litigation and prevent adverse events in the future. Evidence-based medicine is a significant element within the clinical governance agenda and QOF. Interestingly, Goossens et al. (2008) found that doctors were more willing to adopt a guideline when it's based on good evidence. Nurses' adoption scores were higher if they were interested in the subject of the guideline; both felt that if they had higher management support then it would make implementation easier, entrenching it within the organisational governance agenda. Therefore in the case of QOF it can be noted that successful attainment of targets relies on a whole-team approach.

The QOF is part of the General Medical Services Contract (DoH, 2003) which is a voluntary incentive scheme for General Practitioner (GP) practices in the UK. It contains groups of indicators based on evidence from NICE and the National Service Frameworks (NSF). Organisational domains such as the significant event audit can be useful tools for the practice team to re-evaluate and reflect on challenging situations. Table 1.3 highlights examples of the type of event that practice teams may face in response to the Harold Shipman Clinical Audit (DoH, 2001), which recommended mechanisms to enable the health service to detect and learn from adverse events. The Department of Health report in 2000 – An Organisation with a Memory – also suggested regular performance management, i.e., appraisal in order to safeguard the public.

Most of the situations contained within Table 1.3 can prove challenging to the whole practice team. A review is best performed within a confidential, safe and supportive environment with a no-blame culture. The whole point of this is to learn and develop as a group, to look at the events that led to the situation and to analyse processes and decision-making errors, with the aim of preventing a recurrence of the same issue at a later date. An additional outlet for complex issues may include the practitioner taking the scenario to clinical supervision, which is discussed next.

TABLE 1.3   QOF Indicator: Education

QOF indicator – Education: The practice has undertaken a minimum of twelve significant event reviews in the past three years:

- Any death occurring in the practice premises
- New cancer diagnoses
- Deaths where terminal care has taken place at home
- Any suicides
- Admissions under the Mental Health Act
- Child protection cases
- Medication errors
- A significant event occurring when a patient may have been subjected to harm, had the circumstance/outcome been different (near miss).

(DoH, 2003)

Clinical supervision

Clinical supervision is included within the Domain 6 competencies for Advanced Practice (RCN, 2010): Monitoring and Ensuring the Quality of Advanced Health Care Practice '– *Engages in clinical supervision and self evaluation and uses this to improve care and practic*e.' The aim of clinical supervision is to provide a broad range of reflective and critical analysis of care given, in order to ensure quality patient services. Importantly, it should not be confused with other supervisory activities such as appraisal or performance management. The significance of clinical supervision for advanced practitioners is to use it as an aid to the decision making process within a safe, supportive environment which is embedded within the clinical governance agenda. The RCN (2003) describes it as being client centred and focused on safeguarding standards of client care; organisations also benefit from clinical supervision because it can provide:

• Improved service delivery
• New learning opportunities
• Risk and performance management
• Systems of accountability and responsibility.

For practitioners, this can give enrichment of day-to-day practice; provision of celebration, encouragement and advice for complex professional and clinical issues. Clinical supervision can be organised in a variety of ways such as:

• One-to-one supervisor (Supervisor-Supervisee)
• Group Supervision (Supervisor-Supervisees)
• Peer Group Supervision (Dual Roles: Supervisors/Supervisees).

Ideally you should choose the scenario which is most appropriate for your learning and developmental needs. Nevertheless even if you are lucky enough to have this activity funded by your employer you may not be able to choose your preferred method or your preferred peers. However it can still be a useful instrument for reflection, facilitating empathy and cohesion within a team. Example 2 demonstrates how friction within the team could have hindered clinical decision making in primary care.

Example 2

This session was attended by four practice nurses, one ANP, four GPs and an external facilitator. A GP initiated the discussion by saying she felt under pressure and irritated by frequent interruptions to her consultations from the nurses. She felt that because of this the care she was providing in her consultations was compromised.

The main response to this was the practice nurses reminding the GP that often they were dealing with complex decisions that needed timely advice – for example, issues surrounding titration of insulin; exacerbations of COPD/Asthma; prescribing or social issues. The other GPs and the ANP did not support the GP. In fact they were glad to be interrupted if it prevented an error being made by another practitioner or having to make another appointment for the same patient with them.

This scenario threw light on some uncomfortable issues. It was acknowledged by the participants that the doctors were also asking for advice; not just from each other but from the nursing team especially in areas such as chronic disease management. The workload for the on-call GP was unbalanced; causing stress to be experienced by the GP and compromised care to patients.

Following discussion, it was agreed that asking for and providing help is one of the most important things a practitioner must do. The GP recognised the value of the clinical input from the nurses and that their questions were just as valid as the doctors. The nurses appreciated the pressures that the GP was under and were able, in the end, to view this situation sympathetically. Everyone was forced to review their rationale for disturbing consultations, raising awareness of boundaries and timely interruption. The clinical supervision session was a confidential meeting; most of the partnership was present. Subsequently the on call arrangements were reviewed and revised as a result of this session.

Activity 3

Do you or would you engage in clinical supervision if your employer or organisation did not value its effectiveness? If not valued, think of ways in which you could still engage in the process with your peers.

Used in the right environment, clinical supervision can provide APs with an opportunity for lifelong learning, facilitate insights into clinical practice, develop new knowledge and provide an opportunity for innovation in practice within the clinical governance framework. It can bring into play memories, incidents or clients which may have been affected by personal judgement; helping to shift perspectives, be open to new ideas and understand that personal actions were either correct or could have been improved. Many advanced practitioners are fortunate to access clinical supervision within the workplace; however, if they do not they may find it useful to forge their own peer group support externally, using strict ground rules with issues such as patient and group confidentiality. These sessions could take the form of lunchtime meetings if time is available. Otherwise evening meetings, social networking such as Facebook, conference calls and electronic blogs may be alternatives.

Evidence-based decisions

In order to build a cognitive toolkit and develop skills for improved decision making, APs need to have knowledge of critical appraisal and use the best available evidence in order to enhance the patient outcome and quality of life. Domain 6 of the Competencies for Advanced Practice (RCN, 2010) expects the ANP to monitor current evidence-based literature in order to implement quality care. The characteristics of the best research evidence are:

> Clinically relevant research which invalidates previously accepted diagnostic tests and treatments and replaces them with new ones that are more powerful, accurate, more efficacious and safer.
>
> (Sackett et al., 2000:1)

Experience can provide a false sense of certainty and is of little help when faced with a situation you have not previously encountered. A good decision from an evidence-based perspective is one that successfully integrates the following four elements:

- Professional Expertise 'Know-How' Knowledge
- The Resources Available
- The Patient's 'Informed' Values
- The Research Knowledge or 'Know-What' Knowledge.

Professional expertise – 'know-how' knowledge

This is the ability to use your clinical skills, knowledge and judgements to guide decision making. For example, a research paper may suggest treatment which really is not suitable for your patient. It takes confidence, knowledge and experience to realise this and to become an effective advocate for and with your client.

The resources available

This could include your relationship and ability to communicate effectively with colleagues and employers and to consider whether they are open to change and innovation within your department. Consider example 2. How would the practitioners have overcome introducing innovation in practice if this situation had not been rectified? Consider the following in relation to resources:

> Will the cost of the treatment outweigh the benefits? Many GPs are now anxious that barriers to prescribing non funded drugs within the NHS will now fall to them. By 2013 GPs will have to make these choices for their own consortia and justify decisions to their patients.
>
> (DoH, 2010)

Are you able to access IT and find summaries from sources you can trust i.e., systematic reviews, Cochrane Library and NICE guidance? Can you decide whether this information holds relevance for your practice or client group?

Even if you are able to access this information, it is not easy to analyze a paper. Do you have support to access the skills needed to proceed? Can you network with your colleagues to make this easier?

The patient's 'informed' values

It is important when considering concordance with treatment or medication regimes that you listen and understand your patient's ideas, concerns and expectations. Table 1.4 uses the STEPS acronym (Pegler and Underhill, 2005) to help you decide whether an intervention would be appropriate for your client. Once you have made sense of this for yourself you will be in a better position to pass this on to your patient.

The research knowledge – 'know-what' knowledge

The huge amount of information at our fingertips makes it tricky to navigate, but in order for Evidence Based Medicine to inform your decision making processes it is important to understand the following:

• The difference between a randomised controlled trial and an observational study or case report
• What longitudinal or cohort studies involve
• How meta-analysis is constructed

TABLE 1.4 The STEPS Test

Safety: Remember that only limited safety information is available from prospective clinical studies and Randomised Controlled Trials. Safety data from real-life comparison studies may be more useful as these will reflect the patient population.

Tolerability: Rates of withdrawal of interventions in clinical studies can be an indicator of whether interventions have effects that will influence compliance.

Effectiveness: Consideration should be given to whether the drug/intervention works in the real world.

Price: All costs should be considered including the extra costs of titration and regular monitoring.

Simplicity of use: Frequency of administration, ease of delivery and use can mean the difference between compliance and non compliance.

(Pegler and Underhill, 2005)

- What methods were used to gain information and was the sample size adequate?
- Was there any bias in funding, questionnaires or a conflict of interest?
- How to assess the validity of different sources of evidence (refer to Table 1.5).

TABLE 1.5 Hierarchy of strength of evidence used in grading recommendations in NICE clinical guidelines (strongest to weakest)

1a	Evidence from systematic reviews or meta-analyses of randomised controlled trials.
1b	Evidence from at least one randomised controlled trial.
11a	Evidence from at least one controlled study without randomisation.
11b	Evidence from at least one other type of quasi-experimental study.
11	Evidence from non experimental descriptive studies, such as case control studies.
1V	Evidence from expert committee reports or opinions or clinical experience of respected authorities.

(Sackett et al., 2000:172)

Conclusion

Clinical decision making is probably what separates practitioners from advanced practitioners. It is difficult to define how clinical decisions are made, and a lot depends on the experience of the clinician and their familiarity with the situation. However, it is clear that up to date current knowledge is essential in making good and safe clinical decisions. However, clinical decisions are never simply about the facts. A good clinical decision is one that balances the research, patient preferences and resource awareness with clinical expertise that is supported by a robust clinical governance framework.

References

Bench-Capon, T. (1990) *Knowledge Representation*. London: Harcourt Brace Jovanich.

Benner, P. and Tanner, C. A. (1987) How expert nurses use intuition. *American Journal of Nursing*, 87(1): 23–31.

Berger, M. (1984) Clinical thinking ability and nursing students. *Journal of Nursing Education*, 23(7): 306–8.

Bloom, B.S. (1956) *Taxonomy of Educational Objectives*. Boston: Allyn and Bacon.

Botti, M. and Reeve, R. (2003) Role of knowledge and ability in student nurses' clinical decision-making. *Nursing and Health Sciences*, 5(1): 39–49.

Burman, M. E., Stepans, M. B., Jansa, N. and Steiner, S. (2002) How do NPs make decisions? *The Nurse Practitioner*, 27(5): 57–64.

Council for Healthcare Regulatory Excellence (2009) 'Advanced Practice: Report to the four UK health Departments'. Available from: http://www.chre.org.uk (accessed 14/06/2011)

Department of Health (1993) *A Vision for the Future. Report of the Chief Nursing Officer*. London: Department of Health.

—— (1998) *A First Class Service: Quality in the New NHS*. London: Department of Health.

—— (2000) *An Organisation with a Memory*. London: Department of Health

—— (2001) *Harold Shipman Clinical Practice 1974–1998 A Clinical Audit commissioned by the Chief Medical Officer*. London: Department of Health.

—— (2003) *Delivering Investment in General Practice: Implementing the New GMS Contract*. London: Department of Health

—— (2010) *Equity and excellence: Liberating the NHS*. London: Department of Health

Elstein, A. S. and Schwartz, A. (2002) Evidence base of clinical diagnosis. *British Medical Journal*, 324: 729–32.

Goleman, D. (1998) *Working with Emotional Intelligence*: New York: Bantam

Goossens, A., Bossuyt, P. and de Haan, R. (2008) Physicians and nurses focus on different aspects of guidelines when deciding whether to adopt them: an application of conjoint analysis. *Medical Decision Making*, Jan/Feb. 28(1):138–45.

Haynes, R. B., Devereaux, P. J. and Guyatt, G. H. (2002) 'Physicians' and patients' choices in evidence based practice: evidence does not make decisions, people do.' BMJ. 324:1350

Jones, F. P. (unknown) Available from: *Quotationsbook.com/quote/13383/* (accessed 14/06/2011)

KSF (2005) 'Knowledge and Skills Framework'. Available from: http://www.skillsforhealth. org.uk/about-us/resource-library/doc_view/509-skills-for-health-learning-design-principles. raw?tmpl=component (accessed 14/06/2011)

Mandin. H., Jones, A. and Woloschuk, W. (1997) Helping students learn to think like experts when solving clinical problems. *Academic Medicine* 72(3): 173–79.

National Institute for Health and Clinical Excellence (2011) Available from www.nice.org.uk (accessed 14/06/2011)

Nursing and Midwifery Council (2005a) *Implementation of a framework for the standard for post registration nursing. Agendum 27.1December 2005/c/05/160* Available from: http://www. nmc-uk.org/Get-involved/Consultations/Past-consultations/By-year/The-proposed-framework-for-the-standard-for-post-registration-nursing-February-2005/ (accessed 14/06/2011)

NHS Knowledge and Skills Framework (2005a) Available from: http://www.dh.gov.uk/ en/Publicationsandstatistics/Publications/PublicationsPolicyAndGuidance/DH_4090843 (accessed 14/06/2011)

Offredy, M. (1998) The application of decision making concepts by nurse practitioners in general practice. *Journal of Advanced Nursing*, 28(5): 988–1000.

Peglar, S. and Underhill, J. (2005) Evaluating promotional material from industry: an evidence based approach. *The Pharmaceutical Journal*, 274: 271–74.

Royal College of Nursing (2003) *Clinical Supervision in the Workplace. Guidance for Occupational Health Nurses.* London: Royal College of Nursing.

—— (2010) *Advanced Nurse Practitioners – an RCN Guide to the Advanced Nurse Practitioner Role, Competencies and Programme Accreditation.* London: Royal College of Nursing.

Sackett, D. L., Richardson, S. W., Rosenberg, W. and Haynes, R. B. (2000) *Evidence-based Medicine: How to Practice and Teach EBM.* London: Churchill Livingstone.

Skills for Health (2010) *Proven role templates for a skilled and flexible workforce.* Available from: http://www.skillsforhealth.org.uk/rethinking-roles-and-services/proven-role-templates-for-a-skilled-and-flexible/ (accessed 14/06/2011)

Thompson C. and Dowding D. (2002) *Clinical Decision Making and Judgement in Nursing.* London: Churchill Livingstone.

Chapter 2　**Consultation Skills**

Victoria M. Lack

Introduction

The ability to carry out a competent consultation involves more than the capacity to take an accurate history, perform a physical assessment, make a differential diagnosis and devise a plan of action. It requires the ability to gain an understanding of what the patient needs and wants from the encounter, an awareness of hidden agendas and the competence to conclude the consultation when both patient and clinician are in agreement about a plan of action, and for both to understand what is going to happen next. It is also about being safe and using current evidence-based practice. In this chapter the nature of the consultation is investigated and ways of ensuring a successful consultation, with best possible outcomes for patient and clinician, are discussed.

Learning outcomes

At the conclusion of this chapter you will be able to:

- Discuss consultation theory with reference to a selection of recognised models
- Consider ways in which to improve consultation skills
- Explore ways in which to evaluate consultation skills in practice.

Background

The ability to assess a patient's problems and needs is an essential skill in all health professions (McGee, 2009). Interestingly, however, the Royal College of Nursing (RCN) competencies for advanced practice do not specifically refer to 'consultation skills' (RCN, 2010). Domain 2 is concerned with the nurse-client relationship and its competencies include the ability to establish partnerships, 'mutual trust' and a sense of 'being there' for the patient. It is presumed that consultation skills must be incorporated in these competencies since they are not specifically mentioned.

The RCN guidelines for accreditation of Advanced Nurse Practitioner (ANP) courses necessitate that the content of ANP programmes include the following:

- Therapeutic nursing care
- Comprehensive physical assessment of all body systems across the life-span
- Health and disease, including physical, sociological, psychological, cultural aspects
- History-taking and clinical decision-making skills/clinical reasoning
- Applied pharmacology and evidence-based prescribing decisions
- Management of patient care
- Public health and health promotion
- Research understanding and application
- Evidence-based practice
- Organisational, interpersonal and communication skills
- Accountability – including legal and ethical issues
- Quality assurance strategies and processes
- Political, social and economic issues
- Leadership and teaching skills
- Advanced change management skills
- Leading innovation.

(RCN, 2010)

Again, consultation skills are not explicitly mentioned. What are included are history-taking, clinical reasoning skills and physical assessment skills. McGee (2009), in a discussion regarding advanced assessment and differential diagnosis, says that interpersonal competence is an essential component of the meeting between two people. McGee doesn't call it a consultation: the health professional must be able to engage directly with the patient as a person as well as being able to take a detailed history (McGee, 2009). McGee goes onto describe in detail the process of history-taking. However, it would seem that there is more to a consultation than interpersonal skills and the ability to take a complete history. Maguire and Pitceathly (2002) indicate that doctors with good consultation skills are able to identify patients' problems more accurately; patients are better satisfied with the process and have a greater understanding of their condition. Patients are therefore more likely to follow the recommended treatment. It also appears that good consultation skills increase job satisfaction for the practitioner (Maguire and Pitceathly, 2002). It could be extrapolated from this that any health professional with good consultation skills will perform better, but at present it seems that it is not something that is considered as an essential competency of advanced level practice, for nurses at least.

When a master's programme, for the preparation of ANPs in primary care, started at a university located in a large city in England, there were sessions provided in a physical assessment module that were dedicated to taking a comprehensive history. The remainder of the physical assessment module was based around assessment of various body systems. It was assumed that it was enough to teach the nurses about systematic history-taking in order to be able to start an effective consultation. After all, the nurses were experienced and had been taking histories for years; they knew all about communication skills: active listening, open and closed questions, positive body language and so on. However, what appeared to be the case is that nurses learn about just that: communication skills and then maybe systematic history-taking. They do not necessarily learn how to put the two together into an effective consultation. In clinical visits to student advanced practitioners, it became apparent that the course was not facilitating development of effective consultation skills. An example illustrates this point:

Example 1

A student in the health assessment module was assessing a lady who had come for a quick urgent appointment at the General Practitioner (GP) practice. She was complaining of diarrhoea and abdominal pain. The student took an adequate, if lengthy, history, performed a competent physical assessment and discussed the diagnosis as being probable gastro enteritis; probably not a surgical cause, and advised the lady to increase fluids, eat bland food as wanted and to come back if the symptoms worsened. This was all fine; except the lady already considered that she had gastro enteritis and knew what to do about it. She was not worried about the abdominal pain being of a surgical cause. She was in fact concerned about when she could return to work as she was a catering assistant and had been sent home. It was easy for me to see from my privileged position as an outside observer that the lady was not getting the consultation she wanted or needed. Not because the nurse was doing the wrong thing, but because she did not understand what the lady wanted, as the lady had not been given an opportunity to tell the nurse what she wanted.

Most information around consultation skills are written for doctors, and mostly for GPs, as they have been aware for many years of the importance of consultation skills. However, much of what is discussed in the training of GP registrars is transferable to the advanced practitioner in primary or secondary care. In order to see where the nurse may have gone wrong in the example above, it may be useful to look at a couple of models of medical consultations.

The traditional medical model focuses on tasks to be done:

The patient says what their symptoms are;
The clinician asks questions and examines the patient;
The clinician says what the problem is and pronounces a treatment;
The patient goes away.

(Moulton, 2007:14)

This describes what happened in example 1, but the needs of the patient were not met. A different approach is the model examined by Roger Neighbour in his well-known book 'The Inner Consultation' (Neighbour, 2005). Neighbour discusses five checkpoints in the process of the consultation:

Connecting with the patient – The clinician acts, listens and asks questions in such a way that the patient feels able to talk and discuss the issue.

Summarizing – This is where the clinician summarizes what the patient has said and checks that they have understood.

Handover – This is where the clinician discusses with the patient what is to be the plan of action and both agree on what will happen next.

Safety netting – The clinician ensures that there is nothing that has been left out from the consultation; no other symptoms or factors which need to be considered. The clinician also ensures safety by discussing with the patient what to do if things to do not go as expected and there is a worsening of the symptoms and or condition.

Housekeeping – This check point is very important for the clinician. This is essentially about time for the clinician to consider whether they have done everything as well as can be done; that all bases have been covered. It is also time to recover from a bad consultation and ensure that you are fit to go on and deal with another patient.

In example 1, the nurse did not effectively connect with the patient as she did not understand fully why the patient had come. In addition, the nurse did not effectively summarize her impression of the situation to the patient. If the nurse had summarised her impression, there would have been an opportunity for the patient to come back and say that actually she was not worried about gastro enteritis, but about when she could return to her job.

Neighbour (2005) also discusses the concept that most GPs will have 'two heads' during the consultation and that there will be an inner and an outer consultation taking place; hence the name of his book. The organiser 'head' is the intellectual part of the brain which takes on the 'managerial' role in the consultation. The second head, the 'responder' keeps track of emotions, sensations and feelings during the consultation and will respond to more emotional cues from the patient. Neighbour (2005) indicates it is desirable to have both 'heads' on during the consultation so both practical and emotional needs of the patient will be addressed.

David Pendleton et al. (2003) wrote *The Consultation: An Approach to Learning and Teaching* in 1984, which provides another well known model of consultation theory and practice. In *The New Consultation* published initially in 2003, Pendleton et al. provide a simplified model for the consultation:

- Understand the problem
- Understand the patient
- Share understanding
- Share decisions and responsibility
- Maintain the relationship
- . . . and do all this within the allocated time!

(Pendleton et al., 2003)

The above list is quite self-explanatory, and emphasises the need for a shared understanding between patient and clinician, as does Neighbour's (2005) model. Broken down a little further, there are tasks to be accomplished at each stage of the above list. In order to understand the patient's problem the clinician needs to understand its nature and history, its aetiology and its effects on the patient. The clinician also needs to understand the patient: their experience of the illness or problem and also the effects it is having on the patient and their life. It is also important to explore what ideas they have about their illness, and what expectations they have from the consultation. The second task, according to Pendleton et al. (2003), is to achieve a shared understanding about the problem and about options for management according to the best evidence available. Task three then is to help the patient choose the most appropriate course of action according to the options open to them. Task four is to agree on the appropriate responsibilities and agree targets, monitoring and follow up. Finally, the clinician needs to consider potential problems that the patient may face and risks factors that may impede a positive outcome to the consultation. The clinician should try to encourage the patient toward as good health as is possible through health promotion advice. This model focuses on understanding the patient and their problem; something that was not done in example 1. Had the nurse been able to understand why the patient had consulted in example 1 and what expectations the patient had from the consultation, there may have been a more mutually satisfactory ending achieved in a quicker time.

Both Neighbour's (2005) and Pendleton et al.'s (2003) models have much to inform the advanced practitioner. Pendleton et al.'s summary of tasks is very simple to understand and the model is very warm and compassionate. Neighbour's practical description of 'checkpoints' in the model is very helpful in setting up a comprehensive consultation style. In addition, the housekeeping task of Neighbour's model is essential in maintaining efficacy and preserving the well-being of the practitioner.

Developing consultation skills allows the clinician to implement a range of styles to suit individual patients and circumstances. This can be beneficial to the clinician and patient (Pendleton et al., 2003). More specifically, the way a consultation is carried out affects the patient's adherence to treatment plans. Patients prefer, and do better, when they are involved in the medical decision making process. There is evidence that long-term outcomes are affected by doctors using a more patient-centred approach to the consultation. It also appears that patients are less likely to sue when they feel they have been understood and respected whatever the outcome of care (Pendleton et al., 2003).

An effective consultation style is also important for job satisfaction amongst clinicians. Understanding how to make consultations a more comfortable process for clinicians and patients can decrease stress (Maguire and Pitceathly, 2002). It is also more interesting to be curious about the process: patients may consult for the same problem many times in a week, but being able to see and understand and work with the nuances that patients bring to the problem makes the work more interesting and satisfying.

Consider ways in which to improve consultation skills

Nurses and other healthcare professionals (HCPs) have traditionally worked with people where the diagnosis or intervention is already known. Practice nurses for example have usually known the content of their surgeries; Ms B is coming for a blood pressure check, and Ms C for a pill check, etc. In these situations, effective consultation skills are still desirable as patients often have another agenda and may require help on another topic. However, it is perhaps not essential that nurses and other HCPs who are not working at an advanced practice level are able to tease out the real reason behind the attendance, as in most cases it is already stated, and if this wasn't the case the patient could always re-consult the GP. In any case, nurses are usually not taught formal consultation skills, leaving them to muddle through and learn from experience how to get 'to the bottom' of what the patient needs and wants. In the world of advanced practice however, it is essential that nurses and other HCPs are able to do this; as the patient often does not come with a diagnosis, and the nurse/HCP needs to be able to find out what is causing the problem before sending them home. It is also desirable for the reasons described above: to improve patient adherence and for job satisfaction. In this section some techniques which can be used to improve consultation skills will be discussed: some adapted from existing models and incorporating the experience of contemporary APs.

First of all it is important to let the patient tell their story. How you begin a consultation is very important. What do you normally say? Maybe you have been taught to start with a bland opening comment such as:

'Hello Mrs B, how are you today?

How can I help you?

What have you come for today?'

These may seem quite neutral openers and an invitation for the patient to tell their story, but the patient may actually answer the question which may not be what you want. For example: in answer to the last question, the answer might be: 'Well, I've come for antibiotics', which is a difficult way to start off. Moulton (2007) suggests saying almost nothing, except for a polite:

'Hello, have a seat.'

The patient is then obliged to make a start with no directing from the clinician. The patient may then say what they've actually been rehearsing to say in the waiting room. Try it!

Of course some people will not say anything. In this case, an opening question is necessary. But even then the silence may be important. Neighbour (2005) says that the first part of the consultation is the only part that the patient has much control over: they tend to make an opening statement, which he calls the curtain raiser e.g., 'I only just made it here in time.' Then the patient may say what they want: 'I just want a repeat prescription of Ventolin'. By asking an initial question, Neighbour thinks you may cut off the curtain raiser which may be important in finding out the mood of the patient and how the patient will behave during the consultation.

Once the patient has said their 'gambit' they will usually go on to expand on this (Pendleton et al., 2003). They will usually talk for up to 90 seconds, at the end of which you may know most of the things which are important to the history and have a good understanding of the patient's perspective. It is very tempting to interrupt the patient at this point, to want to clarify a certain point. Try not to interrupt, but to make encouraging noises or say throw away lines such as 'I see' or 'go on'. You may be surprised at the end how much you know and how little clarification is needed. Pendleton et al. (2003), also write about the clinician needing to have curiosity about the patient: it is important to care why the patient is there and to want to understand the problem. Having curiosity will facilitate listening rather than talking. Of course, the clinician needs to be curious and to listen but also be able to find out what is causing the problem and have the skills and knowledge to make an accurate diagnosis and treatment plan. This requires a new way of history-taking, where the traditional skills of taking a problem-orientated history are blended with an empathetic approach and a desire to fully understand the patient and why they are there (Pendleton et al., 2003).

At this point, the clinician should have 'connected' with the patient, to use Neighbour's (2005) language. There should be a shared understanding of the problem and the patient's responses to it. Pendleton et al. (2003) suggest asking the following questions in order to ascertain that shared understanding has been achieved:

> Do I know significantly more about the patient than before the consultation?
>
> Was I curious?
>
> Did I listen?
>
> Did I explore the patient's ideas, concerns, expectations, and the effects of the problem?
>
> Did I acknowledge the patient's viewpoint?
>
> Did I make an acceptable working diagnosis?
>
> (Pendleton et al., 2003:54–55)

Below is an example of how a potentially important diagnosis was nearly missed as the above questions were not answered.

Example 2

A 17-year-old boy came with his father for an out of hours (OOH) evening consultation. The presenting symptom written on the computer screen was 'abdominal pain; seen by GP this afternoon'. The boy walked into the room, not in obvious distress, and sat down. His father came in behind. The boy was not an easy historian and found it difficult to describe the location, features and intensity of the pain. The nurse, feeling that this was a bit of a waste of time, as the boy had only seen his GP that afternoon, questioned him about what the GP had said and done. The boy found it difficult to remember but said something about lansoprazole and coming in with a stool sample to the OOH. The nurse asked the boy if he had done as the GP suggested and he said he hadn't. The nurse then asked why he had returned so soon after being seen, and he said because the pain had not got any better. At this point the nurse was irritated, as the boy had not done as instructed but had come back anyway. He did not say that the pain had worsened. The nurse nearly sent him away, but felt should probably examine him again.

Upon examination it turned out that the boy was very tender over the right Iliac fossa, had rebound tenderness, a positive Rovsing's sign and was admitted for suspected appendicitis. His C Reactive Protein (CRP) was 159. Considering the above example with respect to the questions above, the nurse's mistakes are easy to see. Partway through the consultation the nurse did not know much more about the patient than before the consultation: such as why he had re-attended and why he had not followed the original GP's advice. The nurse was not curious as she was irritated that the boy had attended at all, and therefore did not listen. The nurse certainly did not explore the patient's ideas, concerns, expectations, and the effects of the problem or acknowledge the patient's viewpoint as she was concentrating on her own viewpoint which was that this patient was wasting her time. Therefore the nurse very nearly did not come to an acceptable working diagnosis. It was only on physical examination, where the severity of the problem was obvious, that the nurse realised that the boy was in fact a very stoical young person who knew that he was unwell and had made a sensible choice in returning for further advice as his abdominal pain was worsening. The above experience made the nurse feel uncomfortable that she had not treated the boy and his father with respect. As a result she nearly missed an important diagnosis as she did not feel it was necessary to examine him as he had so recently been examined.

Pendleton et al.'s (2003) questions can be a helpful reminder during a consultation to ensure that the clinician makes a valid attempt to discover the real presenting problem and reach a satisfactory diagnosis. Pendleton suggests that the questions should be on our desks as a constant reminder.

Activity 1

Use Pendleton's (2003) questions to evaluate two or three consultations. Do they help to identify your strengths and weaknesses in those consultations?

Another vital aspect of the consultation, albeit a perhaps very obvious one, is that the clinician needs to have adequate knowledge and skills. It is all very well being nice and caring, but if the clinician cannot make all attempts to find out what the actual problem is, using their diagnostic skills as well as communication skills, the patient will not benefit. More about this will be discussed in the next chapter on diagnostic reasoning, but it is also worth mentioning here as it is so important.

Example 3

There were several students from the local Walk in Centre (WiC) on one of the 'First Contact Courses' at a London university. The students had already been working at the WiC for a while, but had never undertaken a formal history-taking and physical assessment course. Part way through the course, the lead nurse from the students' WiC phoned up wondering 'who had put the fear of God in them.' The lead nurse went onto say that previously the nurses had been happy to see patients presenting with ostensibly 'simple problems' independently, but now were asking a second opinion on everything. The lead nurse was curious to know why this change had taken place.

This phenomenon of nurses (and other healthcare practitioners) apparently taking a step backwards in their clinical work is not unusual, and is probably necessary. It is described by Moulton (2007) as the move through four stages:

* Unconscious incompetence
* Conscious incompetence

- Conscious competence
- Unconscious competence.

The nurses in the above example had moved from unconscious incompetence in their work at the WiC, where they were unaware that their actions could lead to adverse consequences, to conscious incompetence, where they realised that for example, seeing someone with an ear infection, could be a manifestation of a more serious illness. They realised they were unable to tell the difference. This is obviously a necessary step. It has been the case in recent years that nurses have taken on 'first contact' roles for which they are not equipped, as the WiCs and other open access centres have been set up. Many nurses have been placed in situations where they have been seeing, diagnosing and treating patients without the necessary knowledge or assessment skills to make them safe practitioners. In this case, it is necessary for the nurses to 'unlearn' their often self-taught skills and knowledge, realise there is a vast amount to learn, and start again from the beginning. They will then be able to assimilate the new knowledge along with their previous knowledge into a new found conscious competence.

For example, a nurse who has not undergone an advanced practice course may not know all the reasons why someone may have a headache. They may be quite happy to recommend some simple analgesia and send the patient away. Of course, the vast majority of the time there will be no problem and the patient will go away happy and the headaches will go away. However, nurses who have completed first contact courses should know the 'red flags' associated with headaches and how to exclude them, and to refer on if they cannot exclude them. A headache could be temporal arthritis, meningitis or a space occupying lesion. Chances are it probably isn't, but it might be. The clinician newer to an advanced practice role who has undertaken comprehensive training, and has practiced under supervision, will probably be able to discern a 'worrying' headache from a probably normal headache, and be able to live with and mitigate against the small but present possibility that they could be wrong. The clinician then has achieved conscious competence and will be a safe practitioner. It may take them more time to see each patient, they may take longer over each stage of the consultation process, refer to more resources and discuss with colleagues, but they will be safe. Eventually the clinician, if they continue to learn and develop, will be able to recognise and understand potential complications sooner and will have achieved unconscious competence. At this stage, several stages of the consultation process can be blended or missed out as the clinician will recognise a familiar situation. Students working with experienced clinicians often complain that their mentors do not undertake a full history and examination as they have been taught to do. The experienced clinician does not need to, but the students must not copy them as they do not have the experience to 'cut corners': conscious competence must be learned first.

Of course even experienced clinicians will see patients who baffle them from time to time, and then they should realise their incompetence and seek help as appropriate. It is essential as advanced practitioners that we are able to recognise our areas of competence and incompetence and to work within our areas of competence.

In primary care, and to a lesser extent in secondary and tertiary care, there is always an element of risk taking. In General Practice, and in a patient's home, the clinician normally lets the patient go home, or leaves the patient at home, having made a calculated decision that the patient will not deteriorate and will not require urgent medical attention. It is not common in General Practice or in a person's home to have sophisticated testing equipment available, so much is left to the traditional history-taking and examination skills of the clinician. Of course, there is also risk with discharging patients from Accident and Emergency Departments, Outpatient Departments or from a ward. Pendleton et al. (2003) write about sharing decisions and responsibility whereas Neighbour (2005) writes about safety netting. These are two slightly different approaches to the end of a consultation.

Moulton (2007) indicated her first GP trainer told her that out of 20 patients in a morning surgery, 19 will probably have a trivial problem where it doesn't really matter what you do or don't do, so long as you don't cause them active harm. The 20th patient will have something wrong with them. The problem is working out which patient that is. Sometimes it will have been impossible to have predicted which patient with minor symptoms turns out to have a major problem, so it is essential to have a 'safety net' for both patient and clinician to ensure as far as possible that patients do not fall too far.

Moulton identifies 3 safety nets:

> Tell the patient what you think is wrong and what you expect to happen
>
> Tell the patient how they would know if you are wrong
>
> Tell the patient what they should do then.
>
> (Moulton, 2007)

Neighbour (2005) postulates a good test of whether your safety net is adequate is when you come to write it down. This should be in the Plan. If you are unable to document answers to the three questions above according to what you told the patient then you probably did not explain clearly enough.

Example 4

A mother came into the WiC with a 5-year-old child. The child was slightly miserable, but eating, drinking and playing. The temperature and heart rate were slightly elevated and the child's tonsils were red and enlarged, but there were no worrying features. The clinician diagnosed tonsillitis without marked systemic upset and advised antipyretics and fluids. The mother agreed with the diagnosis and plan. The clinician also advised the mother that the child would probably be feeling better within 3 or 4 days and should be better within a week. The clinician told the mum to bring the child back to the GP if the fever went over 39 and/or did not settle with paracetamol/ibuprofen. The mother should also come back or contact OOH if the child had difficulty swallowing fluids, started vomiting or developed any other new symptoms. She should go to Accident and Emergency if the child started drooling, developed a non-blanching rash or had difficulty breathing.

The above may seem quite a lengthy end to consultation, but can be delivered quickly. A ready-made or customised patient information leaflet could also be used. It is difficult to get the balance right of not wanting to worry the patient/parent, but to give them enough information to be able to respond to worrying symptoms quickly. Most patients with a sore throat do not develop quinsy or septicaemia, but occasionally it does happen. It is also important for your defence: if you have documented clearly that you told the patient what to do if an urgent situation presents itself, then the responsibility is with the patient to carry out that action. Finally, it is useful, especially with children, to tell the parents to come back if they are worried. It may be difficult to consider every possibly symptom that may be a cause for concern, and often parents may have a feeling rather than objective evidence that something is not right.

Activity 2

Choose several consultation notes to review against Moulton's (2007) checklist for 'safety netting'. To what extent did you provide the information she suggests should be given? How can you ensure that this information is provided?

Finally, it is essential that clinicians take care of themselves in order that they can best care for others. This is Neighbour's (2005) 'housekeeping' checkpoint and is concerned with stress prevention. Neighbour says the housekeeping checkpoint is reached when one patient has left the consulting room and the next has not yet come in. He defines a key question to ask before getting on with the next patient:

> Am I in good condition for the next patient? If not what do I need to do to prepare myself? Then do whatever it takes to prepare.
>
> (Neighbour, 2005:224)

Example 5

> Mrs Davis came to the WiC with her daughter complaining of shooting pains down both legs which were getting worse. After a lengthy consultation it was apparent that Mrs Davis had type II diabetes which was poorly controlled and may be contributing to the sensation in her legs. What was also apparent was that her sugar level needed to be brought down soon, in order not to risk an episode of non-ketotic hyper-glycaemia. After some reflection, I decided that a same day appointment with the practice would be appropriate as Mrs Davis was not acutely unwell and did not want to be referred to the hospital. I called the General Practice, and was told there were no same day appointments left. I then asked to talk with a GP or nurse. This involved waiting for a call back from the Practice. This is a difficult situation as the call back could be immediate or after a lengthy interval. I asked the patient to wait in the waiting room while I completed a referral letter, by which time the practice still had not rung back. I could see the queue in the WiC was lengthening and I decided to bring in the next patient. Unfortunately the next patient was also complex, and I felt unable to concentrate on this patient as I was wondering what to do if the practice phoned back while the new patient was still in the room. The GP did ring back after some time, and I had to ask the patient to leave the room so I could discuss details with the GP. I felt I did not hand over the diabetic patient very well and also did not manage the subsequent patient well as my mind was in two places.

Example 5 is a common situation and one which is difficult to resolve. Within reason, as long as you expect the call or response to be soon, then it is better to wait than to see another patient. There may be some other task that you can do in the meantime which requires less concentration. It may be a good time to get a cup of coffee – as long as you know you will not miss the call!

Housekeeping is also about the bigger picture of the organisation of consultations. How much time do you have for appointments or visits? Is it enough? Are you often running late? How many times do you get interrupted when trying to talk to or examine someone? Do you have a pager or mobile which is switched on? Does the IT system work well or do you waste time trying to 'get into' certain programs? Does the printer work? Do you have the equipment you need to hand? All of the above questions are certainly factors which can cause stress to patients and yourself and are factors that you should try to sort out. If you have ten minutes for a consultation and always overrun by an hour by the end of the morning, then this is not helpful to anyone. It is much better to be realistic and have patients, when you are running late, be seen by another clinician who is not stressed.

Activity 3

What are the major factors that affect your ability to concentrate on the consultation when you are with a patient? Which of these factors do you have the ability to change and how could you work towards changing them?

Evaluation of consultation skills in practice

Since nurses are not traditionally taught consultation skills, we do not traditionally evaluate them. In contrast, GP registrars have for a number of years undertaken a rigorous training in consultation skills. The Royal College of General Practitioners (RCGP) views effective consultation skills as very important. These skills are assessed in the MRCGP exams (RCGP, 2007). The framework for the assessment resembles the structure of consultation models and is demonstrated in a 15-minute video presentation. The GP registrar must:

- Discover the reason for the patients attendance
- Define the clinical problem(s)
- Explain the problem(s) to the patient
- Address the patient's problem(s)
- Make effective use of the consultation.

(RCGP, 2007)

In order to pass, it is necessary to demonstrate each pass criterion four times in a total of seven consultations. Some of the pass criteria are concerned with safety: for example in the clinical problems sections the student needs to ask sufficient questions to exclude a pulmonary embolism in a person presenting with shortness of breath. Others are more concerned with consultation skills per se. For example in order to discover the reason for the patient's attendance, the doctor should use silence, minimal encouragers, reflecting, echoing and encouragement to 'go on'. A merit can also be awarded in this section if the doctor is seen to respond to cues which facilitate a deeper understanding of the problem.

The use of video is used by GP registrars both to develop consultation skills and for these skills to be assessed in practice. It is a method which is highly effective, and encourages students to practice and develop competency in consultation which is then demonstrated to examiners. It would be, and is in some advanced practice programmes, a very good tool for developing skills and assessment of skills for advanced practitioners. However, it is important to use video consultations in the correct way. Most of us can cringe with embarrassment at being seen on film, especially when we are trying to demonstrate a skill which is not second nature. Pendleton et al. (2003) set out guidance for feedback of video consultations in their book which have come to be known as Pendleton's rules. These are in essence:

> The student in the consultation should be given the opportunity to give feedback first and discuss the positive points raised. It is essential that positive points are discussed first.

> The student may then say what they feel would have improved their performance.

> The rest of the observing group can then give feedback, but must start with the positive.

> The group can now provide constructive feedback of areas identified for possible improvement by the student. It is these points that can be taken in a negative fashion. Therefore the group facilitator needs to ensure this does not happen and that the comments are not regarded as destructive.
> (Garala, 2007)

It may be that for advanced practice students who are not familiar with this method of assessment, that individual feedback with a mentor is preferable to begin with. The Consultation Assessment Tool (CAT) is a tool used by GP trainers to evaluate taped consultations and is very applicable for Advanced

Practitioners' use in evaluation both during and after training. The tool asks questions about the process and outcome of the consultation. This can be found on page 15 of the following document:

http://www.rcgp-curriculum.org.uk/PDF/curr_2_The_GP_Consultation.pdf

Video consultations are a very good method of developing effective consultation skills and also for maintaining and improving on them. Other methods which are also effective are role play of real or given consultations and one-to-one or group discussions where practitioners bring consultations to discuss. Patient satisfaction questionnaires can also be used to ascertain the efficacy of the consultation from the patient's perspective (RCGP, 2007). All of these are less intrusive and worrying for the student than the traditional sitting in with the student, which has a place in learning and assessment but which can fail to give a true reflection of the ability of a clinician due to the clinician being nervous during the assessment.

Conclusion

The consultation has been a neglected area of advanced practice, perhaps because it has been assumed that nurses and other HCPs are already experienced practitioners and know how to manage effective consultations. However, it is argued in this chapter that this assumption is wrong. As advanced practice involves seeing more complex patients where the diagnosis may be unknown or uncertain this assumption can also lead to unsafe practice. There is much written on consultation skills for GPs. Subsequently advanced practice nurses and other HCPs can make much use of the experience and knowledge obtained by GPs in this area and adapt this information for use in their own practice.

References

Garala, M. (2007) Aids to Learning, In R. Charlton, (Ed.), 2007, *Learning to Consult*. Oxford: Radcliffe Publishing.

Maguire, P. and Pitceathly, C. (2002) Key communication skills and how to acquire them. *British Medical Journal*, 28th September, 325(7366): 697–700.

McGee, P. (Ed.) (2009) *Advanced Practice in Nursing and the Allied Health Professions (3rd Edition.)* Oxford: Wiley-Blackwell

Moulton, L. (2007) *The Naked Consultation*. Abingdon: Radcliffe

Neighbour, R. (2005) *The Inner Consultation*. Abingdon: Radcliffe.

Pendleton, D., Schofield, T., Tate, P. and Havelock, P. (1984) *The Consultation: An Approach to Learning and Teaching*. Oxford: Oxford University Press.

—— (2003) *The New Consultation: Developing Doctor – Patient Communication.* Oxford: Oxford University Press.

Royal College of Nursing (2010) *RCN Competencies: Advanced Nurse Practitioners.* London: RCN Publishing.

Royal College of General Practitioners (2007) *The General Practice Consultation.* Available from: http://www.rcgp-curriculum.org.uk/PDF/curr_2_The_GP_Consultation.pdf (accessed 14/06/2011)

Chapter 3   **Planning Care**

Ruth Walters

Introduction

The aim of this chapter is to explore the use of planning care in promoting health and well-being by empowering patients and encouraging shared decision making within the context of advanced clinical practice. The challenge facing healthcare professionals (HCPs) in planning effective care with patients must not be underestimated. The process requires the utilisation of a range of skills and competencies. Non-medical prescribing is now embedded within advanced clinical practice for many disciplines and along with planning care is included in the discussions within this chapter.

Learning outcomes

At the conclusion of this chapter you will be able to:

- Critically examine the role of care planning in your area of work
- Identify the range of skills required for successful care planning
- Develop knowledge in enabling a holistic care planning approach
- Develop skills in helping patients to set realistic goals.

Enabling concordance with healthy lifestyles choices, encouraging participation in appropriate screening programmes and achieving adherence to medication and treatment regimes is a goal to which all health care professionals aspire. Patient-centred care planning can provide the foundation on which to build therapeutic relationships, increase knowledge and develop the skills and competencies required by patients to achieve this goal. There is growing evidence that effective self care is as important as medical intervention in managing diabetes (Department of Health [DoH], 2007a, 2008; Healthcare Commission, 2007). The importance of the development of the ability to self manage is evident in the example of the patient with diabetes, who spends on average three hours per year in contact with HCPs (DoH 2007b). The individual lives and manages their diabetes within the society and culture shaped and informed by their own, family, and peer knowledge, beliefs and skills for an overwhelming majority of their life. What is true for diabetes may also be true for management of other long-term conditions.

In considering care planning for advanced HCPs it is important to understand that aspects of advanced clinical practice will differ according to the profession, specialty and place of care delivery. Planning care should form the basis of patient centred care whatever aspect of treatment or care one is proposing to enable or deliver. This chapter will include a range of case studies to provide examples of care planning in advanced clinical practice in a variety of settings.

Background

Care planning is contextualised according to the specialty and environment in which the care delivery is planned and must be responsive to the needs of the individual. Using the example of care planning for patients with long-term conditions, there is a significant consensus that it is the process of collaborative and supportive care planning rather than the produced care plan which is important (National Diabetes Support Team, 2008; National Health Service [NHS] Modernisation Agency, 2005).

Many services and organisations will have templates and documents for written care plans and these vary in their aims and objectives. For the purposes of this chapter a care plan is simply defined as the product of a collaborative process. In the instance of a consultation for a minor ailment, this could be the outcome of a discussion between patient and healthcare provider that certain simple self care measures be adopted and a review planned if there is no improvement in symptoms within a time frame. Alternatively, it could be a complex written document held by both the HCP and the patient detailing agreed specific goals and actions, some of which may be long term goals such as weight loss, smoking cessation and/or concordance with complicated medication regimens.

Irrespective of the complexity and format of the plan, the defining characteristics of care planning should remain the same in order to achieve the anticipated outcomes. The plan must be:

- Holistic
- Patient centred
- Owned by the patient and be in a format which can be easily accessed and understood
- Goals must be realistic and achievable.

The advanced practitioner will be required to draw on a range of skills and competencies to enable successful care planning. There are a range of tools in the form of competency frameworks which can help define standards, guide professional development and enable reflection on practice. The Royal College of Nursing (RCN, 2010) Domains of Competence for Advanced Nurse Practitioners outlines key competences for this professional group and it has been noted that a number of these competencies are evident in standards expected of other professional groups when examining advanced practice within their specialty (Cox, 2010).

TABLE 3.1   Domains of Competence for Advanced Practice

Domain 1:	Assessment and management of patient health/illness status;
Domain 2:	The nurse/patients relationship;
Domain 3:	The education function;
Domain 4:	Professional role;
Domain 5:	Managing and negotiating healthcare delivery systems;
Domain 6:	Monitoring and ensuring the quality of advanced healthcare practice;
Domain 7:	Respecting culture and diversity.

(RCN, 2010)

The National Prescribing Centre (NPC) has also developed competency frameworks for nurse, pharmacist and allied HCP prescribers (NPC 2001; NPC 2004; NPC 2006). Many of the competencies in the NPC frameworks can be aligned with those in the RCN (2010) framework but are applied more specifically to the prescribing issues relevant in advanced clinical practice. These provide useful frameworks for those wishing to develop skills and review the need for continuing professional development in non-medical prescribing. The RCN Domains 2 and 3 will be used to focus a critical discussion in relation to care planning; however it should be noted that the other domains in this framework also discuss relevant skills and competencies and must also be considered.

Prerequisites for planning care

Good communication is essential in establishing the effective and meaningful relationship with patients and clients necessary to negotiate a successful plan of care. Domain 2 of the RCN competencies focuses on the nurse/patient relationship, see Table 3.2.

TABLE 3.2 Competencies in Domain 2

Domain 2: The nurse/patient relationship

- Creates a climate of mutual trust and establishes partnerships with patients, carers and families;
- Validates and checks findings with patient;
- Creates a relationship with patients that acknowledges their strengths and knowledge, and enabling them to address their needs;
- Communicates a sense of 'being there' for the patient, carers and families and provides comfort and emotional support;
- Evaluates the impact of life transitions on the health/illness status of patients, and the impact of health/illness on patients' lives (individuals, families, carers and communities);
- Applies principles of empowerment in promoting behaviour change;
- Develops and maintains the patient's control over decision-making, assesses the patient's commitment to the jointly determined plan of care, and fosters personal responsibility for health;
- Maintains confidentiality, while recording data, plans, and results in a manner that preserves the dignity and privacy of the patient;
- Monitors and reflects on own emotional response to interaction with patients, carers and families and uses this knowledge to further therapeutic interaction;
- Considers the patient's needs when bring closure to the nurse-patient relationship and provides for a safe transition to another care provider or independence.

(RCN, 2010:14)

The following case study will be used to critically discuss elements of the nurse/patient relationship domain and identify their relevance in care planning and ensuring effective practice.

Example 1

S is a 49-year-old woman who has type 2 diabetes and hypertension; both diagnosed four years previously. S last attended a diabetes review at the practice ten months ago with another HCP. At the last consultation a review date had been set for three months as her glycosylated haemoglobin (HbA1c) was considered high and a change in medication dosage made. At this consultation it was noted that S stated that she was taking her medication as prescribed. Since this time S has requested two repeat prescriptions (both issued for a one month supply); the last request being four months previously. A review of the notes indicates that prior to the consultation ten months ago, S had only been prescribed a total of 90 days' supply in the previous 12 months. S had attended an appointment with a health care assistant who had taken blood tests and recorded Blood Pressure (BP) and weight two weeks ago. S is attending now for an annual review. Her test results show an increase in the HbA1c level and her BP remains elevated. S has lost 5kg in weight and her current BMI is 28. S received a letter explaining these results in the mail one week before she attends for her care planning consultation.

During the consultation, S reveals that she has not been taking any of the medication at all. S requested the prescriptions and obtained the medication which is still in a cupboard at home. S states that this is because she has read the patient information leaflet and is scared of the side effects listed.

Create a climate of mutual trust and establish partnerships with patients, carers and families

Given the limited time usually available, the advanced HCP must be able to establish quickly good communication with an individual. In the example of S, where S is suffering from a long-term condition, it is also essential that the HCP gain the trust of others whom S may wish to include in planning her care, such as family members. These significant others will have a considerable influence on S's future actions and behaviours. Mutual trust also implies that the HCP trusts the patient and requires an environment in which the patient will feel able to accurately inform the HCP about her concerns, identified problems, current lifestyle and medication use. S had stated at a previous consultation that she was taking her medication but a review of the records shows only a supply of ninety days medications in a twelve month period. This raises questions for the HCP about S's understanding of frequency and dosage of the medications and her motivation for concordance with the regime.

In order to elicit an accurate answer to these questions S must feel able to trust the HCP. There is a wide range of verbal and non-verbal communication skills which can facilitate the establishment of trust and some of these are discussed later in this chapter. The HCP must remain conscious of the social and cultural differences between patients when utilising these skills (Thompson, 2010).

An important part of establishing a successful therapeutic relationship with S will be establishing a no-blame culture to enable her to feel that she will not be judged or made to feel guilty about her lack of adherence to medication. It is also essential that the HCP takes care not to create an environment which encourages patients to 'please' the HCP by reporting complete concordance where none exists.

Create a relationship with patients that acknowledge their strengths and knowledge, and enable them to address their needs

Creating a partnership with a patient and enabling shared decision making is viewed as essential in effecting improved health outcomes for patients in all aspects of care and treatment (Clyne et al., 2007; Coulter, 2009; NICE,

2009a; NICE, 2007). Patients present with a wide range of personal experiences, knowledge and beliefs and in order to influence any of these, the HCP must first understand pre-existing conditions. In the first example, S presents as an individual with 'uncontrolled' long-term conditions according to the biochemical outcomes measures suggested in national guidance (NICE, 2009b). At this stage the HCP does not have any knowledge of S's understanding of these diagnoses and implications for her health. The use of open questions will help to elicit a broad outline of the situation and the use of a closed question to focus in can be helpful. For example the open question:

'What do you understand about how what you eat can affect diabetes?'

Such a question could help the HCP to gain an understanding of S's perceptions about her self-efficacy and self-knowledge as well as giving an understanding of her knowledge base. This could then be followed up with:

'So you are finding the system of food labelling confusing. Have you had any information about food labels in the past?'

Reflecting on the conversation can ensure that we have gained an accurate understanding of what we have been told and ensure that we don't allow any misconceptions to arise which may influence our future actions and negatively impact on the relationship with the patient.

S was noted to have lost weight at the review. She may raise this herself but the use of a focussed closed question can provide the HCP with further understanding of any factors which may have affected this.

'I notice that you have lost weight. Was this something you planned?'

The outcome of the response to this question can help direct the HCP to potential future education and support. If the weight loss is the result of a planned change in behaviour by S then acknowledgement of her success and further support to continue will be useful. If the weight loss is not planned and S is unaware of any changes which would have triggered this then this might indicate a need for a different plan of care entirely, including an assessment of risk for co-morbidities.

Activity 1

Think of a question that you use frequently in your area of work. Is it an open or closed question? Consider if this is the most appropriate type of question and consider what rationale you have for using this type of question.

Active listening

The use of open or closed questioning will help our understanding and enable the development of our relationship *only* if we are willing to listen to the answers. Active listening can be challenging, particularly in a situation where time is limited. The HCP may be thinking ahead to the next question or may be distracted by interruptions. It is important that not only do we gain the information required, but that the patient feels that their words are being understood and valued in order to further develop the relationship of mutual trust. Active listening involves showing a response to what is being said, this can be verbal or non verbal but care must be taken to ensure that the focus remains with the speaker.

Verbal signals

The use of phrases such as 'go on' and 'I see' can ensure that you do not interrupt or draw attention away from what the patient is expressing but can indicate to the patient that you are interested and actively listening to their story. Niven (2006), also discusses the use of reflecting back and paraphrasing as tools in active listening. The use of these can also help us to prompt further information and to check the accuracy of our understanding.

Non-verbal signals

The HCP must be aware of the non-verbal signals that are unconsciously sent. Body posture, head movements and eye contact all indicate to the person with whom we are interacting our level of interest in what they are saying and can also convey approval (or disapproval). The use of non-verbal signals can encourage the patient to continue talking and reveal more information or conversely can effectively draw a conversation to a premature end.

Monitor and reflect on your own emotional response

Every practitioner works within a frame of reference influenced by previous experiences and personal beliefs. Understanding and acknowledging these beliefs and attitudes can enable the advanced HCP to avoid adopting judgmental attitudes with patients who may choose a course of action which is not concordant with our view of the world. S has made a conscious decision not to take the medication and has not trusted others with this knowledge. It is essential that the HCP responds in a non-judgmental way to S's revelation, taking an open approach that allows her to voice her concerns and doubts about any aspect of her care including the prescribing of medication. Any attempt to blame S will be detrimental to the relationship and is unlikely to result in increased adherence. The HCP should use verbal and non-verbal skills to demonstrate an understanding of the complex reasons for her behaviour.

It is estimated that between 35% and 50% of medications prescribed for long-term conditions are not taken as prescribed (NICE, 2009a). There may be a wide range of reasons for non-adherence which may be multi-factorial. In S's example we see clearly see a failure to agree a *shared* plan of care initially – the HCP issued a prescription for an increased dose of a medication which S had already made a decision not to take. In addition there is no evidence of support for adherence. For instance, a plan to review after one month to check for side effects or to answer queries.

Activity 2

Think of a situation where a patient or client has not taken a medication as prescribed. Make a note of how you felt about this, how this influenced subsequent care and what actions you took. Consider what could have been done differently and how this would have influenced the outcomes.

The care planning process

'Care plans' have been employed in health care for many years but in the past they have often been led by clinicians and the focus has been on the production of a written care plan to direct the team of HCPs. In recent years there has been increasing evidence that shared decision making and emphasis on the *process* of care planning results in greater patient satisfaction and is more likely to achieve the goals identified in the final agreed care plan (Clyne et al., 2007; Coulter, 2009; NICE, 2007).

The Year of Care Model (National Diabetes Support Team, 2008) outlines the following domains which must be addressed in order to ensure a holistic approach to care planning:

- Emotional
- Social
- Clinical
- Behavioural
- Knowledge and health beliefs.

The RCN framework describes the advanced practitioner role in the area of knowledge and health belief in Domain 3: The Education Function (RCN, 2010).

TABLE 3.3 Competencies in Domain 3

Domain 3: The Education Function

Timing

- Assesses the on-going and changing needs of patients, carers and families for education based on a) Need for anticipatory guidance associated with growth and the developmental stage. b) Care management that requires specific information or skills. c) The patient's understanding of their health condition;
- Assesses the patient's motivation for learning and maintenance of health-related activities using principles of change and stages of behaviour change;
- Creates an environment in which effective learning can take place.

Eliciting

- Elicits information about the patient's interpretation of health conditions as part of the routine health assessment;
- Elicits information about the patient's perceived barriers, supports, and modifiers to learning when preparing for patient's education;
- Elicits the patient's learning style to facilitate an appropriate learning approach;
- Elicits information about cultural influences that may affect the patient's learning experience;
- Enables patients, by displaying sensitivity to the effort and emotions associated with learning about how to care for one's health condition;

Enabling

- Enables patients in learning specific information or skills by designing a learning plan that is compromised of sequential, cumulative steps, and that acknowledges relapse for the need for practice, reinforcement, support and re-teaching when necessary;
- Enables patients to use community resources when needed;
- Communicates health advice and instruction appropriately, using an evidence-based rationale.

Providing

- Negotiates a jointly determined plan of care, based on continual assessment of the patient's readiness and motivation, re-setting goals, and optimal outcomes.

Negotiating

- Monitors patient's behaviours and specific outcomes as a guide to evaluating the effectiveness and need to change or maintain educational strategies.

Coaching

- Coaches the patient by reminding, supporting and encouraging, using empathy.

(RCN, 2010:15)

Timing

Example 2

M is a 37-year-old Bengali man who attends a practice requesting help with stopping smoking. He has been smoking for 20 years and reports smoking 15 cigarettes a day. This has increased over the years from five cigarettes per day initially. The nurse calculates this as equivalent to 13 pack-years. M says he has to give up as he has been made redundant recently and financially he cannot afford to keep buying cigarettes. M's wife attends with him and says she is worried about his health as her father suffered from COPD and died aged 57 years.

M attempted smoking cessation six months previously and used nicotine replacement patches. He stopped smoking completely for a period of two weeks and then restarted which M feels was due to stress at work

Assess the patient's motivation for learning and maintenance of health-related activities using principles of change and stages of behaviour change

The process of any change in behaviour begins with the identification of a need or desire to change. The identification may arise from within an individual, be prompted by a person with significant influence such as a close friend or colleague or may come from a healthcare worker. In the case study given, M indicates that the trigger for his deciding to attempt behaviour change is the financial cost of continuing to smoke. Whatever the trigger any attempt to coerce or persuade an individual to change behaviour is unlikely to succeed and may in fact damage the therapeutic relationship. The stages of change theoretical model developed by Prochaska and DiClemente (1986) outlined five stages of change. These are:

Precontemplation – the patient is not contemplating any change within the next six months
Contemplation – there is an intention to change within the next few months
Preparation – the patient is making plans to change in the near future
Action – the stage during which the patient is making specific behavioural changes
Maintenance – this period is estimated to last from six months to five years.

This was later updated to include a sixth stage – **termination** – a term used to describe a stage whereby the individual no longer has any desire to relapse regardless of any mitigating factors. Using this trans-theoretical model can help understand M's progress in his attempts to stop smoking; his relapse and preparation to try again. It can also help us to understand the need for support during the action and maintenance stages.

Motivational interviewing (MI) is an approach which can be used to explore factors which could motivate and potential barriers to change with an individual. MI aims to utilise the patient's own goals and system of values to stimulate a desired change in behaviour. A basic tenet of the approach is that the motivation to change is elicited from the patient and not imposed; the skilled motivational interviewer will gain an understanding of the individual's motivating factors and reinforce these whilst challenging any barriers which are elicited. In M's case, this could involve discussing the financial cost of smoking and calculating a monthly or annual figure to reinforce the benefit to the family finances. The use of support and reinforcement to empower the individual to change is central to the approach and the patient's belief in their self efficacy is essential.

The main components of MI can be viewed as:

- Empathy
- Allowing the patient to resist and regarding resistance or denial as a sign that the practitioner is assuming a readiness to change which doesn't exist
- Supporting self-efficacy.

Greaves et al. (2010)

A Cochrane review of randomised controlled trials using MI in smoking cessation was cautious in its analysis of effectiveness due to variations in study quality but concluded that it may help smokers to quit (Lai et al., 2010).

Eliciting

Example 3

A need was identified to increase the uptake of childhood vaccinations in a multicultural inner city area as levels of uptake were insufficient to assume herd immunity. It was assumed that the controversy regarding MMR vaccination was largely responsible for a decline in confidence in the programme and the low uptake of vaccination. A network of four GP practices planned an event incorporating entertainment activities for children, experienced nurses to discuss immunisation with parents and offer immunisation if required. A presentation was prepared on MMR vaccination and delivered twice during the day. The expert delivering the presentation was also available for discussion with parents. All parents of children who had not completed a full vaccination schedule received an invitation to the day.

The issue of assessing need in an individual is discussed earlier in this chapter. The HCP may also be called upon to assess need and plan care for a group of individuals. In this case study the need was identified using data which showed levels of uptake insufficient to assume herd immunity. An assumption was made that the controversy regarding MMR vaccination was largely responsible for a decline in confidence in the programme and the low uptake of vaccination. This assessment was based on anecdotal evidence from HCPs in the area and discussions in the media.

The MMR expert delivered the presentation which was well received. During discussions with parents, the expert received several queries about polio vaccination from parents who had recently emigrated from eastern Europe. It emerged that the live polio vaccine is still used in some countries and concerns had been raised about polio vaccine related morbidity.

In this example, the HCPs had made assumptions about the cause of low uptake for vaccination which provide to be, at least partially, inaccurate. We must take care to ensure that our assessment is thorough and encompasses a wider evidence base than can be gained from personal experiences. In this situation the influences gained from peers within a cultural group had caused parents to make a decision not to vaccinate their children. The need for use of public health information and epidemiological data is identified in Domain 1 of the RCN competences (RCN, 2010).

Enabling

Example 4

A, a 35-year-old woman attended a family planning clinic requesting the combined oral contraceptive pill (COC) as she had previously been prescribed this elsewhere. The HCP undertook a full assessment encompassing previous medical history, a gynaecological history, family history, BP, weight, BMI and smoking history. The HCP used the information gained to assess the suitability of this method for A and decided that it was contraindicated.

This example requires a careful discussion with A so that A will understand why the method is contraindicated. Initially the HCP must assess how much A understands about the drug and possible risk and benefits. It is also important to gain an understanding of A's previous experiences with contraception and her need for this contraceptive therapy. Open questioning around previous discussions with HCPs would provide insight into this area.

> The HCP informs A that the method is contraindicated and she must stop taking it. A is very upset. She has had problems in the past with dysmenorrhea which was relieved by the COC. A feels that this issue was not raised by her previous GP. The HCP feels defensive, but is sure that she is right, and that to prescribe the COC would not be in the patient's interests. A immediately leaves the consultation feeling frustrated that she cannot obtain the treatment she wishes to have.

This outcome clearly demonstrates the poor outcomes which can be expected when the HCP fails to gain an understanding of A's 'need' for the COC. In this case study had the HCP approached the situation more sensitively and provided options for other more suitable methods of contraception, the outcome may have been very different. A would have been enabled to make a decision regarding the form of contraception. In this situation, the HCP must also watch for A's emotional response. Defensive behaviour is likely to result in the deterioration of a therapeutic relationship.

Activity 3

Using the above case study consider how the HCP could have approached this situation and what techniques could have be used to improve the outcome so that A could have been enabled to make an appropriate decision regarding contraception.

Providing

Example 5

> Mr K is a 65-year-old man who was diagnosed with type 2 diabetes two years ago. He attended two weeks ago and had blood and urine tests, BP, weight and a foot check. At this consultation the HCP discussed Mr K's lifestyle in terms of diet and exercise patterns and had referred Mr K to a local exercise scheme. Mr K had received the results of the assessment in the post a few days before the care planning consultation. The results show that Mr K has gained weight and his HbA1c has increased over the past 6 months.

The Year of Care model being used in this context provides Mr K with information about the results of parameters used to determine the current state of control of his diabetes. Traditionally the HCP would hold this information and give whatever the HCP felt appropriate to the patient when the patient attended the consultation. The use of traditional a medical model ensures that the clinician remains in control and leads to a disempowered patient who has insufficient information to make informed decisions. Receiving the information in advance also allows Mr K time to reflect on possible contributing factors.

> The HCP asks Mr K if there are any questions he has about the results letter.

Mr K asks some questions about the exact nature of the kidney tests and he demonstrates a good understanding of the answers.
The HCP must ensure that an individual has a good understanding of any relevant literature including the results letter. The use of written literature must be approached sensitively. An individual may find it difficult to acknowledge that they cannot read or write and in some spoken languages there may not be a written language.

> The HCP asks Mr K whether he feels any of the results should be improved.

Asking Mr K to identify his priorities will help to ensure that any of his concerns are addressed first and enables the HCP to develop an understanding of what goals Mr K might wish to address. The results of an ensuing discussion will allow the HCP to identify key areas of educational need and a plan can begin to be developed between the HCP and the patient.

The consultation must be adapted to suit not only an individual's communication and learning preferences but must also be culturally relevant and sensitive.

Negotiating

Example 6

> L is a 44-year-old Caucasian woman who was diagnosed with type 2 diabetes seven years ago. L works full time in a career which requires extensive travelling, staying in hotels and entertaining clients. L maintains good control of both HbA1c and glucose levels on monotherapy. L was overweight at diagnosis and has since gained a further 7 kg. Her BMI is now 33. L is unhappy about this weight gain. L attends her local GP practice requesting medication to aid weight loss and after discussion regarding a range of options a plan is agreed to a trial of orlistat medication.

Negotiation requires both parties to understand and share a common goal. If the HCP identifies a need for weight loss but the patient does not view this goal as a priority it is unlikely that any change in behaviour leading to weight loss will occur. In the case of L, she had already identified the goal of weight loss and declared herself ready to address the weight gain. In this case study there will be many contributing elements to the care plan including education and support for learning in knowledge of food types and portion sizes and support for increasing physical activity (perhaps referral to exercise schemes) all of which will require negotiation. A plan may be agreed for L to start walking to work in the morning but if, at review, this goal has not been achieved then clearly a change of approach or goal is required. Perhaps the goal was too ambitious – the walk too far or time consuming; the route may be unpleasant or considered unsafe to walk. Using the skills discussed earlier in the chapter to elicit the barriers can aid in the development of realistic goals.

L has requested medication to help her weight loss and the plan of care agreed includes the use of this drug. The HCP using national guidance discusses target weight loss with L and agrees a review date.

> L attends for review after four weeks and has lost 1kg, which is half the agreed goal. L is disappointed, stating that she feels she had lost more than this but last week she had a family crisis and had less time to plan and prepare meals. L was relying on takeaways and also stopped taking the medication, last week, because of side effects.

The HCP must continually evaluate an individual's motivation and readiness to change. It would be appropriate to reflect back to L the situation and directly challenge her readiness for change. The HCP might say something like:

'So things have been stressful and you have not really been able to keep to the plan. Is this something that is now resolved?'

Coaching

Example 6 continued

L reveals that her younger brother had peritonitis and was very ill. He is now making a good recovery. L says that this was a one-off situation; that everything is resolved and she is ready to try again.

The HCP will empathise with an obviously stressful and traumatic situation. The coaching function describes the use of reminding, support and encouraging. The HCP can use the weight loss, although small, to encourage L and discuss the fact that she had effectively changed her behaviour for a period indicating her efficacy to do so again. The use of this support for self efficacy is consistent with the principles in motivational interviewing discussed previously. The opportunity should be taken to assess the need for further educational needs indentified by L or any barrier encountered. The care plan should be reviewed in terms of the actions and goals and agreed in the light of the previous experiences. Another review date should be identified.

If, however, the situation is ongoing, L must be given the opportunity and space to decide that this is not the right time to engage and a plan could simply be that a review will take place after a period of time and another assessment made of her readiness to change. It is important to remember the earlier discussion about emotional response in this situation. The HCP may feel that there has been a significant investment in time, financial resources in medication costs and effort and feel frustrated at the lack of change. However the HCP must accept that there may be other external influences which bring a stronger imperative and therefore the 'investment' will not yield the desired response at this particular time.

Conclusion

This chapter has used the RCN (2010) and NPC (2001; 2006) frameworks to critically examine many of the skills and competencies required in planning care with patients and has considered the use of skills identified in motivational interviewing. There are many other theoretical models and frameworks which HCPs will find contribute to the development of effective care planning.

Care planning must be a flexible process which accounts for each patient as a unique individual who will require a different approach and will have a different set of goals. Arguably the most important element of the care plan is that both the individual and health care professional are actively working towards common goals.

The use of a care planning process to successfully promote health and well-being is a challenging role and in some areas of practice this will be a team approach contributed to by many practitioners, in others it may only involve an individual HCP, but at the centre must always be the patient.

References

Clyne, W., Granby, T. and Picton, C. (2007) *A Competency Framework for Shared Decision Making with Patients: Achieving Concordance for Taking Medicines.* Staffordshire: National Prescribing Centre Plus.

Coulter, A. (2009) *Implementing Shared Decision Making in the UK.* London: The Health Foundation.

Cox, C. L. (2010) *Physical Assessment for Nurses.* Oxford: Wiley-Blackwell.

Department of Health (2007a) *Working Together for Better Diabetes Care* London: Department of Health.

—— (2007b) *Supporting People with Long Term Conditions* London: Department of Health.

—— (2008) *Five Years On: Delivering the NSF.* London: Department of Health.

Greaves, C., Shepherd, K. and Evans, P. (2010) Motivational interviewing for behavioural change: *Diabetes & Primary Care* 12(3): 178–82.

Healthcare Commission (2007) *Improving Services for People with Diabetes.* London: Commission for Healthcare Audit and Inspection.

Lai, D. T., Cahill, K., Qin, Y. and Tang, J. L. (2010) Motivational interviewing for smoking cessation. *Cochrane Database Systematic Review* 2010 Jan 20th (1).

National Diabetes Support Team (2008) *Partners in Care: A Guide to Implementing a Care Planning Approach to Diabetes Care.* London: Health Foundation.

National Institute for Health and Clinical Excellence (2007) *Behaviour Change at Population, Community and Individual Levels.* London: National Institute for Health and Clinical Excellence.

—— (2009a) *Medicines Adherence.* London: National Institute for Health and Clinical Excellence.

—— (2009b) *Type 2 Diabetes: The Management of Type 2 Diabetes: An Update.* London: National Institute for Health and Clinical Excellence.

National Prescribing Centre (2001) *Maintaining Competency in Prescribing – An Outline Framework for Nurses.* Liverpool: National Prescribing Centre.

—— (2004) *Maintaining Competency in Prescribing – An Outline Framework to Help Allied Health Professional Supplementary Prescriber.* Liverpool: National Prescribing Centre.

—— (2006) *Maintaining Competency in Prescribing – An Outline Framework to Help Pharmacist Prescribers: 2nd Edition.* Liverpool: National Prescribing Centre.

NHS Modernisation Agency (2005) *Good Care Planning for People with Long Term Conditions: Updated Version.* London: NHS Modernisation Agency.

Niven, N. (2006) *The Psychology of Nursing Care (2nd Edition)*. Basingstoke: Palgrave MacMillan.

Prochaska, J. O. and DiClemente, C. C. (1986) Toward a comprehensive model of change. In: W.R. Miller and N. Heather, (Eds). *Treating Addictive Behaviors: Processes of Change*. New York: Plenum Press.

Royal College of Nursing (2010) *Advanced Nurse Practitioners – An RCN Guide to the Advanced Nurse Practitioner Role: Competences and Programme Accreditation*. London: RCN Publishing.

Thompson, K. (2010) Working with individuals and groups: Creating and strengthening relationships. In C. L. Cox and M. C. Hill (Eds), 2010, *Professional Issues in Primary Care Nursing*. Oxford: Wiley-Blackwell.

Section II **Management**

Chapter 4 **Management Theory**

Marie C. Hill

Introduction

The role of the Registered Nurse (RN) and the Allied Healthcare Practitioner (HCP) has changed significantly in the United Kingdom (UK) since the 1990s. For example, RNs, whether in the acute or primary care setting have seen their roles and responsibilities dramatically change more so as a consequence of a change in service provision from the acute to primary care sector. This has lead to an increase in services within primary care and with this a need to examine who provides these services. This has led to new opportunities for RNs to take on roles previously within the domain of a general practitioner (GP). Practice Nurses (PNs) have risen to this challenge and the new General Medical Services (new GMS) contract has led to an increase in the numbers of PNs making them the largest branch of primary care nurses (Macdougald et al., 2001). This role evolvement includes some PNs acquiring advanced skills in assessment, diagnosis and prescribing, whilst others have developed entrepreneurial skills and have become practice partners with their GP colleagues (Derrett and Burke, 2006). Furthermore, RNs in the acute sector have taken on these roles as well as leading on services such as the role of the nurse consultant; again a change in roles once seen as traditionally medically dominated. The introduction of the European Working Time Directive in 1998 initially excluded junior doctors with respect to specifying minimum requirements for working hours and annual leave requirements (Goodling, 2009). However, since 2004 junior doctors are not excluded and it can be argued that this Directive has and will have a significant impact on how new roles are developed for nurses; particularly as the maximum weekly working hours have been reduced to 48 hours as of August 2009 (Goodling, 2009). It can be argued that these changes not only promote the nursing profession, but highlight the career opportunities and different pathways and choices that are now available for RNs. However, newly formed nursing teams with diverse responsibilities bring with them challenges for the advanced practitioner who manages these teams. The aim of this chapter is to explore management in terms of definition and theories of management including their influence on today's organisations.

Learning outcomes

At the conclusion of this chapter you will be able to:

- Explore the various definitions of management and distinguish management from administration
- Understand how management theory has evolved and developed
- Critically appraise the diverse role of the manager
- Explore how the Advanced Nurse Practitioner domains; in particular Domains 5 and 6 can be integrated into management decision making on patient quality care outcomes (RCN, 2008)
- Examine some of the strategies that managers use.

Background

What is management?

A clear cut definition of what a manager is, is difficult to obtain as there is no universally accepted definition of the term management (Cole, 2004). Others have argued that a precise definition is impossible due to the variety of management posts in the workforce (Jones and Jenkins, 2006). Indeed, some writers have debated that there is a relationship between management and leadership:

> Leadership is viewed by some as one of management's many functions: others maintain that leadership requires more complex skills than management and that management is only one role of leadership.
>
> (Marquis and Huston, 2009:31)

However, it is not the intention of this chapter to delineate between leadership and management, as firstly leadership will be explored in detail later in this book and secondly, the focus of this chapter is on management with particular emphasis on advanced practice.

There are a number of definitions of the term management. Some of these are:

> The action or manner of managing
>
> (The Shorter Oxford English Dictionary, 1973:1269)

TABLE 4.1   The management process

1. Planning: Planning functions include determining philosophy, goals and objectives, policies, procedures, and rules; carrying out long-range, intermediate, and short-range planning; fiscal planning; and managing planned change.
2. Organizing: Organizing includes establishing the structure to carry out plans, determining the most appropriate type of patient care delivery, and grouping activities to meet unit goals. Other functions include working within the structure of the organisation as well as understanding and using power and authority appropriately.
3. Staffing: Staffing functions include recruitment, interviewing, hiring and orientation. Scheduling and staff development are additional staffing functions. Socialization of employees is also frequently included as a staff function.
4. Directing: Some management experts place several staffing functions under the directing phase of the management process. However, usual functions listed in this phase are the human resource management functions: that is, motivating, managing conflict, delegating, communicating and facilitating collaboration.
5. Controlling: Controlling functions include performance appraisals, fiscal accountability, quality control, legal and ethical control, and professional and collegial control.

(Marquis and Huston, 1998: 20)

> Management is an operational process initially best dissected by analysing the managerial functions . . . The five essential managerial functions (are): planning, organising, staffing, directing and leading, and controlling.
>
> (Koontz and O'Donnell, 1984
> cited in Cole, 2004:6)

It is the latter definition, in relation to the management process, that finds agreement with writers on the sequence of events in relation to this process (Marquis and Huston, 1998). For example, the planning phase always begins the management process, whilst the controlling or evaluation phase ends it. Marquis and Huston (1998) describe the functions of each phase of the management process in Table 4.1.

In Drucker's (1968) book *The Practice of Management*, it was advocated that questioning the exact functions of a manager's role would shed light on a more precise definition of their role and responsibilities. Mitzberg's (1973) definition of the role of manager contrasts in some respects to that of Handy's who identified the role of a manager as one of involving leadership, administration and resolving or fixing (Handy, 1999). Mitzberg viewed that there were three distinct categories to a manager's role:

- Interpersonal, which is figurehead
- Leader and liaison

- Information, which is monitor, disseminator spokesman and finally, decisional roles which are entrepreneur, disturbance handler resource allocator and negotiator.

(Jones and Jenkins, 2006)

Therefore, the administrative role is but one of the many roles that a manager holds and is not an exclusive role.

In appraising organisational effectiveness of a manager, Mintzberg et al. (1995) viewed that this flowed from the interaction and relationship between several factors, which he described as the 7-S framework. The 7-S that he identified were:

Systems

These relate to the formal and informal procedures of the organisation. For example, budgeting and training.

Style

This relates to how power within a team or organisation is managed. This could be in relation to how managers spend their time and could be symbolic in how the team is perceived as managing their time.

Staff

This is two-tiered. Firstly, it relates to appraisal systems and training initiatives and/or programmes with the latter being formal rather than informal training. For example, attendance at a Higher Education Institution for a formal programme (e.g., A Masters in Business Administration or a BSc [Hons] in Primary Care Practice Nursing).

Skills

This relates to current skills and skills that need to be acquired. The latter being identified as new roles that change and evolve within an organisation or during a mid-term/annual appraisal.

Strategy

This is a key function of any organisation and relates to how the organisation needs to change, be responsive to and adopt its functions in response to external forces. For example, a Health Maintenance Organisation (HMO) in the United States of America (USA) or a Primary Care Trust (PCT) in the UK expanding clinical services in the provision of diabetes mellitus specialist nurses due to higher prevalence and incidence of the disease compared to the national average.

Structure

This is how the tasks are delegated within an organisation or team. There is a very strong association here with the 'Skills' function.

Superordinate goals

The values and aspirations of an organisation or team (Jones and Jenkins, 2006).

Therefore, what is important for any manager, particularly in a health care environment, is an understanding of factors that can influence their team's or organisation's effectiveness.

Activity 1

Consider Mitzberg's 7-S framework. How does this framework fit into the team that you manage or would like to manage? What factors are strengths in the team? What are the areas for improvement? How would you improve these? Can you identify any barriers to change?

The evolution of management theory

The role of the manager is indeed diverse, as the previous pages have shown. How has management theory evolved to enable us to understand management in its present day format? Management theory, as with the definition of management, has not been static and the theory itself has been responsive to change due to societal and organisational structure. The birth and development of management theory has been influenced by other disciplines such as: business, psychology, sociology and anthropology (Marquis and Huston, 2009). Indeed, the theory has evolved over the last hundred years due to the complexity and variety of organisations (Marquis and Huston, 2009). The following will be an overview of the development and changes in management theory with examples from contributors to management theory and how these changes have influenced management in organisations beginning with classical theories to modern approaches to management theory.

It was the beginning of the twentieth century in 1925 when the Frenchman, Henri Fayol, first explored a definition of management and the general principles of management (Cole, 2004). His experiences as a mining engineer and latterly as the managing director of the same company led him to publish his work on management and the identification of fourteen principles of management. These are: Division of Work; Authority; Discipline; Unity of Command; Unity of Direction; Subordination of Individual Interests to the General Interest; Remuneration; Centralization; Scala Chain or the Line of Authority in an Organisation; Order; Equity; Stability of Tenure of Personnel (i.e., a period of time allocated to employees to settle into their new role); Encouraging Initiative and Esprit de Corps or Promoting Teamwork and Collaboration (Cole, 2004). Interestingly, it is Fayol that is first credited with identifying the management functions of: planning; organisation; command; coordination and control (Marquis and Huston, 2009) and which are considered to be the 'foundation stones of modern management' (Burtonshaw-Gunn, 2008:132). Although, it was Luther Gulick in 1937 who expanded on Fayol's functions as identified by the following mnemonic – POSDCRB

- Planning
- Organising
- Staffing
- Directing
- Coordinating
- Reporting
- Budgeting.

(Marquis and Huston, 2009)

In essence, Fayol and Gulick laid the framework for the organisation of both work and people. This formal structure of management theory became known as the Classical Theory of Management.

Unlike Fayol and Gulick, Elton Mayo viewed individuals within organisations as key to achieving organisational effectiveness (Cole, 2004). He was the first of a number of theorists (e.g., Maslow, McGregor, Argyris, Likert, and Herzberg) to form what is termed the Human Relations and Social Psychological School of management theory (Cole, 2004). Mayo's research was undertaken over a five year period at the Hawthorn works of the Western

Electric Company in Chicago. Overall, the research (i.e., from 1924–1936 in five distinct stages) revealed that productivity increased even though improvements in working conditions were taken away and productivity results were similar to the control group who did not have these improvements taken away. The key to the increased productivity was revealed as the legacy of good human relations practice between the employers and the employees (McKenna, 2000). Mayo and his colleagues influenced Abraham Maslow and his research into human motivation, which made a significant impact on developments in management theory during the 1950s–1960s (Cole, 2004). Maslow proposed that the majority of people are motivated by the desire to satisfy specific groups of needs. His theory (i.e., the hierarchy-of-needs theory) is represented by the figure of a pyramid with the more basic 'Psychological needs' forming the base of the structure and the most desirable or highest needs in this figure at the top of the pyramid – 'Self-actualisation'. Maslow's needs were as follows:

- Physiological needs
- Safety needs
- Love needs
- Esteem needs
- Self-actualisation needs.

(Cole, 2004)

Although Maslow's work has been highly influential in understanding human motivation, it has been criticized as being too simplistic in assuming that individuals' needs are standardized. Furthermore, his motivational theory does not take into account cultural and individual differences (Marriner Tomey, 2000). There are a number of other motivational theories, such as Roethlisberger and Dickson; Hezberg; McClelland and Ardrey. Readers are referred to Handy's (1999) book *Understanding Organisations* for further information.

Another influence in management theory emerged around the same period as Fayol. Max Weber, a sociologist, was interested in why individuals in organisations obeyed those in authority. Weber identified three types of legitimate authority that are: traditional; charismatic and rational-legal authority (Weber, 1947). It was the publication of Weber's translated text from *The Theory of Economic and Social Organisation* in 1947 that the term 'bureaucracy' was used to describe a rational form of organisation (Cole, 2004). There are a number of different definitions of bureaucracy. Some are:

- Government by many bureaus, administrators, and petty officials
- The body of officials and administrators, esp. of a government or government department
- Excessive multiplication of, and concentration of power in administrative bureaus or administrators
- Administration characterized by excessive red tape and routine.

(Dictionary, 2010)

Whilst Weber identified the main features of a bureaucracy as in essence bound by rules and regulations, there have been critics of this form of management which is referred to as 'the dysfunctional consequences of bureaucracy' (Carnell, 2007:130). Some of these consequences have been summarised as an over-reliance on rules and structure; relationships are predictable based on the role of the individual leading to rigid conformity to the rules and consequently that change is difficult due to adherence to rigid rules and regulations (Cole, 2004). Regardless of Weber's detractors, his influence on management theory has impacted in 'practically every business and pubic enterprise' (Cole, 2004:25).

Following on from the Human Relations and Social Psychological School of management theory, another school of thought began to emerge in the late 1960s. This new school of thought emerged from the Tavistock Institute of Human Relations in London. It recognised that there was more to organisational effectiveness than human or social factors alone because organisations are a complex mix of individuals, tasks and technology. A new phrase was identified – open social technical system, in which an organisation interacts and is interdependent with its environment (i.e., that environment which is key to the organisation's function/business) (Cole, 2004). What emerged from this new theory was that no one theory could guarantee an organisation's effectiveness; rather management had to select from a number of theories that suited the specific needs of that organisation.

From the open systems theory of management emerged the contingency approach to management. The latter theory viewed that a mixture of management theories could be adapted to an organisation. Handy in *Understanding Organisations* argued against a 'universal formula' or one size fits all theory (Handy, 1999:181). However, he noted that 'most modern theories of organisations are increasingly persuaded of the wisdom . . . of the match of people to systems, to task and environment, of inter-relations between all four' (Handy, 1999:181).

Activity 2

Reflect on your team and/or organisation. Considering the theories of management that you have read about, what is the focus of your organisation? Does the team or organisation focus on task? Is it people focused? Or is it responsive to environmental change (e.g., proactive or reactive)? Do you consider that there are other factors that underpin the management of your team or organisation?

List these factors and consider what the drivers and barriers to change are in relation to your team or organisation.

Domains of practice: addressing management and quality

This section on management theory introduces some of the influences on today's organisations. How does management theory influence advanced practitioners in an ever changing health care environment? To mirror Handy's words, the emphasis surely must be on the match of the individual, their role or task, the environment and the interconnection amongst these factors. How does an advanced practitioner deal with the complex interrelations on a team basis or in the wider organisation to meet the needs of the team and ultimately the organisation? How does an advanced nurse practitioner (ANP) or allied healthcare practitioner (HCP) know they are adhering to the required competencies for management and quality? The framework that will be used as a point of reference in this chapter is the domains relating to management and quality from the Royal College of Nursing (RCN, 2008) document: Advanced nurse practitioners: an RCN guide to the advanced nurse practitioner role, competencies and programme accreditation. The publication of this RCN document was driven by the need to produce a framework to identify the role of the advanced nurse practitioner (ANP); the RCN's revised Domains and Competencies for advanced nurse practitioners in the UK and finally the standards expected from Higher Education Institutions (HEIs) wishing to achieve RCN accreditation for their advanced level practice nursing programmes (RCN, 2008). Domains 5 and 6 are listed as follows:

Domain 5 – Managing and negotiating health care delivery systems

Managing

- Demonstrates knowledge about the role of the advanced nurse practitioner
- Provides care for individuals, families and communities within integrated health care services
- Considers access, quality, efficacy and equity when making care decisions
- Maintains current knowledge of their employing organisation and the financing of the health care system as it effects delivery of care
- Participates in organisation decision-making, interprets variations in outcomes, and uses data from information systems to improve practice
- Manages organisational functions and resources within the scope of responsibilities defined in a job description
- Uses business and management strategies for the provision of quality care and efficient use of resources
- Demonstrates knowledge of business principles that affect long-term financial viability of an organisation, the efficient use of resources and quality of care
- Demonstrates knowledge of, and acts in accordance with, relevant regulations for this level of practice and the *NMC Code of Professional Conduct.* The code makes this explicit that practitioners must keep their level of knowledge and skills updated commiserate with their level of practice throughout their career.

(RCN, 2008:17)

Negotiating

- Collaboratively accesses, plans, implements and evaluates care with other health care professionals, using approaches that recognise each one's expertise to meet the comprehensive needs of patients
- Undertakes risk assessment and manages risk efficiently
- Participates as a key member of a multi-professional team through the development of collaborative and innovative practice
- Participates in planning, development and implementation of public and community health programmes

- Participates in legislative and policy making activities that influence health services/patients
- Advocates for policies that reduce environmental health risk
- Advocates for policies that are culturally sensitive
- Advocates for increasing access to health care for all.

(RCN, 2008:17)

Domain 6 – Monitoring and ensuring the quality of advanced health care practice

Ensuring quality

- Incorporates professional/legal standards into advanced clinical practice
- Acts ethically to meet the needs of the patients in all situations, however complex
- Assumes accountability for practice and strives to attain the highest standards of practice
- Engages in clinical supervision and self-evaluation and uses this to improve care and practice
- Collaborates and/or consults with members of the health care team about variations in health outcomes
- Promotes and uses an evidence based approach to patient management that critically evaluates and applies research findings pertinent to patient care management and outcomes
- Evaluates the patients' response to the health care provided and the effectiveness of the care
- Interprets and uses the outcomes of care to revise care delivery strategies and improve the quality of care
- Accepts personal responsibility for professional development and the maintenance of professional competence and credential.

(RCN, 2008:18)

Monitoring quality

- Monitors quality of own practice and participates in continuous quality improvement
- Actively seeks and participates in peer review of own practice
- Evaluates patient follow-up and outcomes, including consultation and referral

- Monitors current evidence-based literature in order to improve quality care.

(RCN, 2008:18)

The following case study is an extract from a nurse consultant's narrative on how she manages and deals with the complexities of her role and that of others within an acute hospital setting.

Case study

The role of the consultant nurse is a complex one and focuses around four key areas of practice:

- Expert practice
- Professional leadership – consultancy
- Education/Training/Research/Evaluation
- Practice and service development.

While this may appear at first a daunting prospect to execute successfully, it is in fact extremely helpful in facilitating continuity of care and the management of health care delivery systems. These four key areas provide an umbrella for the numerous domains and competencies described for advanced nurse practitioners. They too are pertinent when taking into consideration managing a team of highly skilled nursing staff.

Expert practice allows you to talk with authority and provides the opportunity to lead on services within the team and organisation. Drawing on my skills and knowledge enables me to develop strategies of care that will benefit both the local population (applicable to my specialty) and prove to be cost effective for the Trust. This is often carried out in conjunction with key stakeholders from the Trust and the local Primary Care Trust (PCT), and using evidence from national and international initiatives. It also requires the deployment of excellent negotiating skills to ensure mutually acceptable outcomes are achieved.

> 'To keep myself updated within nursing and my specialist area I attend national and international conferences, often attending as a speaker or part of the faculty. This is one way of attending with little or no financial cost and learning from colleges and co-presenters. Anything new learnt can be passed on to the team so that they too get the benefit of my attendance and it maintains my credibility.

My role demands me to work collaboratively with many disciplines each of who often have their own agenda. Overarching, as a nurse, is the priority of patient care, as laid out in the Nursing and Midwifery Council's Code of Professional Conduct. It can be difficult trying to balance the requirements of the Trust verses the requirements of the patient when they differ. Again negotiating skills are essential here.

I believe that managing a team of senior clinical nurses requires me to demonstrate that I possess the skills that I require of them, in order to be an effective leader. It is then that I can appreciate their individual abilities and provide tailored guidance and support. My natural leadership style is 'Participative' as identified through completing the Likert Leadership Style Questionnaire and allows for effective team cohesion. Managing a team of senior clinical nurses requires me to be able to delegate to appropriately experienced members in an attempt to develop staff. This requires me to be visionary in my approach with the team. There are times I may not have all the answers or know the way forward but am willing to experiment and take calculated chances – after all that is how we learn and develop.'

Jane Butler (Nurse Consultant)

Managing people

Managing teams can be complex and challenging as can be seen from the previous narrative. Teams are not homogenous because of the diversity of each team. Therefore, a manager such as an advanced practitioner must acknowledge and work with each individual within the team in order to have a functional team. Hunt (1992) asserts that managers must have a mixture of skills and competencies to manage effectively. These skills and competencies are having interpersonal; knowledge and visionary skills. Yukl (2005) has examined a number of characteristics that effective managers possess. Effective managers:

- Take advantage of reactive activities (i.e. they problem solve; influence others)
- Develop a large network of contacts
- Identify relationships between problems
- Learn from surprises and failures. In this instance the manager is open to suggestions and change
- Are willing to experiment and take chances
- Prioritize problems. This involves examining the trivial problem from the major problem

- Are politically astute. This requires skill in understanding the organisation, its key people and how it works. For example, knowing who has influence in the organisation
- Allow time for reflective planning.

The effective manager needs time to give consideration to plans and how to implement them. Some managers will be creative in how they set aside 'thinking time' to enable them to consider different options to a solution and how best to approach such a solution. There are many reflective models that can be utilised (e.g., Gibbs, 1988; Schon, 1987; Boud et al., 1985). Whatever model is used will depend on previous experience of using a reflective model. However, the use of a model will allow and enable the manager to give consideration to a situation or a problem that they wish to gain further insight into or to resolve.

Clearly, not all managers will have these skill sets. This raises the importance of organisations such as The National Health Service (NHS) to support and develop their managers to their potential. Iles (2006) describes three fundamental rules that a manager needs to follow to manage people effectively. These rules are:

- Clarity on what is expected of the team member to achieve
- Ensuring that the team member has the skills to achieve what is expected to be achieved
- Providing feedback on performance.

These three rules are explored in more detail in the narrative that follows.

Clarity on what is expected of the team member to achieve

This may seem obvious, but the question must be raised: Do all managers engage with their team to ensure that they fully understand what they are expected to achieve in their role? Job descriptions are helpful, but in times of organisational growth and even uncertainly, there can be a lack of understanding by a manager on what they expect their team members to achieve. The role of the manager therefore, is crucial in defining role expectations and particularly how this is communicated. It has been argued that assertive communication is the key to relaying information to others (i.e., the information being relayed is clear and concise) (Sully and Dallas, 2005). It is for the manager to initiate the regularity of meetings with their team members.

Ensuring that the team member has the skills to achieve what is expected to be achieved

An important point for any new manager (i.e., whether they have been promoted in their current organisation or moved to a new organisation) is to individually meet their team members and ascertain what skills they have or indeed do not possess to be able to meet their objectives. For example, an advanced practitioner, who has a partnership in a practice, is keen to increase patient access to services and to reduce waiting times. This ANP or HCP would need to ascertain the level of skills and competence that the other members of the team have. Following individual meetings and meetings with the team, it was identified that there was a need for physical assessment training to be undertaken by one member of the nursing team in order to meet the objectives of increasing services and reducing waiting times. Through the conduction of a needs assessment, other needs for education may be identified such as non-medical prescribing training, in order that the RN has a range of skills and competence to assess, manage and treat clients' as necessary. The ANP or HCP who manages this team would have to consider how they supervise and support the team whilst they are undertaking formal education and additionally when they are applying theory to practice to ultimately ensure that practice is both competent and safe. What may be the most challenging aspect for the ANP or HCP in this instance is that their enthusiasm to implement change must take into consideration the educational needs of the team and importantly the time that this development will require to ensure competency in practice.

Providing feedback on performance

Following on from the two fundamental rules as identified by Iles (2006), the final rule is providing feedback on the team members' performance. This is essential for any manager in order for individuals to progress and achieve their set goals. Annual and mid-term appraisals are a way in which one-to-one feedback on a team member's performance can be given. However, this should not be viewed as the only opportunity to do so. Providing feedback needs to be flexible in how this is undertaken and a manager, such as the aforementioned advanced practitioners, may need to provide this feedback on a regular basis, especially if they are supervising clinical practice. For example, after one of the ANPs or HCPs has undertaken both a physical assessment and non-medical prescribing module, they need to supervise the HCP's effectiveness in assessing clients' in the clinical setting. It can be seen from this example that, an effective manager must be in tune with their team's needs and provide feedback when it is necessary. This will not only enhance their relationship with the team, but promote a functioning team with competent members who are supported and recognised for their contribution to the organisation (Sully and Dallas, 2005).

Activity 3

You are an advanced practitioner who needs to implement a change to service provision within your team. The Chief Executive Officer (CEO) within your organisation has made it clear that an increase in your service provision needs to be 'immediate'. You know the abilities of your team and that any increase in additional services will need training and supervision over at least a period of six months. The other solution is to recruit, but the CEO has not contemplated this and has informed you that 'you must use the skills of your existing team, as we have no money to recruit new staff.'

You are one of the 'rising stars' of your organisation, having won a recent Health Service Journal Award. You are considering applying for a senior management post, which you know will be advertised in the next three months. Therefore, it is essential that you and the team perform well. However, you consider that the CEO's time frame is unrealistic, even though increasing access to health services and monitoring the quality of service are two of the competencies in Domains 5 and 6 respectively for advanced practice.

You do not wish to jeopardize your standing in the organisation because of the forthcoming senior management post. You know there is a solution to this and are going to think of a solution over the weekend. You are scheduled to meet the CEO on Monday morning. How would you approach this problem? You realise that change is inevitable and therefore, you must develop a business plan that is acceptable to the CEO but also to your team. How will you address this to both the CEO and your team?

Conclusion

Today's advanced practitioner, who additionally may have a managerial role, must possess a range of skills that not only include excellent interpersonal skills, but also a critical understanding and indeed an ability to apply **management** theory. This is key to the success of the manager's role in terms of dealing with day-to-day operational issues in the working world. As identified by Handy (1999), there is no universal management theory that meets each organisation's managerial needs, as organisations are not homogenous entities. What is important though is that a manager understands their team and individuals' roles. Ultimately, this may be easier for managers of a small team (e.g., less than 10) in comparison to a team larger than this. However, this will depend on the skills of the manager in how they 'ring fence' time for their team members and, notwithstanding, how they manage their own time. The ANP has a template or framework for how they can meet quality and managerial domains and competences as outlined in the RCN (2008) document. HCPs functioning at an advanced level of practice can use this framework as a point of reference for their own practice. What is not made explicit to the manager working at an advanced practitioner level is how they deal with day-to-day operational issues such as negotiation, influencing, managing change and conflict resolution. The following chapters of this book will show you how to address these issues.

Ultimately, management is giving others the tools and resources to deliver, which is succinctly described by Seden and Reynolds (2003:5) as 'Giving people the ability to do the job that's in front of them.'

References

Boud, D., Keogh, R., and Walker, D. R. (1985) *Reflection: Turning Experience into Learning*. London: Kogan Page.

Burtonshaw-Gunn, S. A. (2008) *The Essential Management Toolbox*. Chichester, West Sussex: John Wiley and Sons, Ltd.

Carnell, C. (2007) *Managing Change in Organisations*. 5th ed. Harlow, England: Financial Times Prentice Hall.

Cole, G. A. (2004) *Management, Theory and Practice*. 6th ed. Australia: South-Western CENGAGE Learning.

Derrett, C. and Burke, L. (2006) The future of primary care nurses and health visitors. *British Medical Journal*, 9th December, 331(7580): 1185–1186.

Dictionary, (2010) Available from: http://dictionary.reference.com/browse/bureaucracy [Accessed 30/09/2010]

Drucker, P. (1968) *The Practice of Management*. London: Pan.

Gibbs, G. (1988) *Learning by Doing: A Guide to Teaching and Learning Methods*. Oxford Polytechnic: Further Education Unit.

Goodling, L. (2009) New Roles for Nurses at Night. *Nursing Standard*, July 8th–14th, 23(44): 62–63.

Handy, C. (1999) *Understanding Organisations*. 4th ed. London: Penguin Books.

Hunt, J. W. (1992) *Managing People at Work*. 3rd ed. London: The McGraw-Hill Companies.

Iles, V. (2006) *Really Managing Health Care*. 2nd ed. Berkshire: Open University Press.

Jones, R. and Jenkins, F. (2006) *Managing and Leading in the Allied Health Professions*. Oxford: Radcliffe Publishing.

Macdougald, N., King, P., Jones, A. and Eveleigh, M. (2001) *A Tool Kit for Practice Nurses*. Chichester: AENEAS.

Marquis, B. L. and Huston, C. J. (2009) *Leadership Roles and Management Functions in Nursing. Theory and Application*. 6th ed. Philadelphia: Wolters Kluwer/Lippincott Williams and Wilkins.

—— (1998) *Management Decision Making for Nurses*. 3rd ed. Philadelphia: Lippincott.

Marriner Tomey, A. (2000) *Guide to Nursing Management and Leadership*. 7th ed. St. Louis, Missouri: Mosby.

McKenna, E. (2000) *Business Psychology and Organisational Behaviour. A Student's Handbook*. 3rd ed. Hove, East Sussex: Psychology Press. Taylor and Francis Group.

Mintzberg, H. (1973) *The Nature of Managerial Work*. New York: Harper and Row

Mintzberg, H. Quinn, J. B. and Voyer, J. (Eds). (1995) *The Strategy Process*. Harlow: Prentice Hall.

RCN (2008) Advanced nurse practitioners: an RCN guide to the advanced nurse practitioner role, competencies and programme accreditation. London: RCN.

Schon, D. A. (1987) *Educating the Reflective Practitioner*. San Francisco: Jossey-Bass Foundation.

Seden, J. and Reynolds, J. (2003) *Managing Care in Practice*. London: Routledge.

Sully, P. and Dallas, J. (2005) *Essential Communication Skills for Nurses*. Edinburgh: Elsevier Mosby.

The Shorter Oxford English Dictionary (1973) *The Shorter Oxford English Dictionary. On Historical Principles*. Volume 1 A – Markworthy. Oxford: Oxford University Press.

Weber, M. (1947) *The Theory of Social and Economic Organisation*. Translated by A. M. Henderson and Talcott Parsons. New York: Oxford University Press.

Yukl, G. (2005) *Leadership in Organisations*. 6th ed. Upper Saddle River, New Jersey: Prentice Hall.

Chapter 5   The Effective Manager: Management skills for the advanced practitioner

Rosa Benato

Introduction

Now you have a good idea of management theory and the differences between management and leadership from the previous chapter. This chapter will help you to develop some specific and more personal management skills through a series of activities. These may not be the skills that you might be expecting to develop as a manager, such as how to effectively manage a budget, or how to carry out an appraisal or a performance review interview. Instead, the focus for this chapter will be on developing your management skills in a more subtle but profound way: developing your own self awareness. You may be wondering how that will help you to become a better manager but by the end of the chapter you will agree that the most important person to get to know well is yourself. The purpose of this chapter is to help you to develop the knowledge, skills and strategies that will give you a realistic and mature confidence to be an effective manager.

Learning outcomes

At the conclusion of this chapter you will be able to:

- Understand the concept of emotional intelligence and identify ways in which emotional intelligence principles can be applied to your own management practice
- Reflect on your communication and management skills
- Develop an insight into your own management skills through reflective practice
- Identify your own strengths and areas for development
- Learn how to identify situations which trigger emotional responses in you and developed strategies to manage these

- Gain an insight into how your actions impact upon others
- Understand the importance of adapting the way you manage according to individual situations.

This chapter will start with some additional management theory. The purpose of including the additional theory is to demonstrate the theoretical basis underpinning the activities and case studies that follow. The chapter will conclude with some key messages for you as a developing advanced level practice manager.

Background

While managers have had a role within the National Health Service (NHS) since its inception, it is only within the last 30 years or so that clinicians themselves have become managers, leading and managing their peers (Salter, 2004). The Griffiths Report (Department of Health and Social Security, 1983) led directly to the current situation of clinicians, trained in their specialist clinical area, taking on the additional duties and responsibilities of managing teams and even entire departments. A delicate balance must be achieved by clinical managers; they must balance the politics of the organisation, with its particular targets and specific demographics as well as current governmental demands. In addition, they must maintain clinical and managerial credibility amongst their peers, continue to enable the consumer-oriented NHS (Iles and Sutherland, 2002; Marsaili et al., 2001), ration increasingly scarce resources and ensure clinical and political accountability (Department of Health, 1998, 2000). This is quite a set of expectations for any manager.

How does an advanced level practice clinical manager successfully negotiate the endlessly changing political landscape and ensure a cohesive, financially prudent service whilst maintaining a close working relationship with the people they manage? What set of specific skills is required to do all this? There are practical skills, often relating to resources, that can be learned on courses, such as how to write a business case, how to manage a budget or how to shortlist and interview. What are far more difficult to learn, far more intangible, are the 'soft' management skills; skills such as managing people, knowing how to deal with conflict or managing change effectively.

How does a manager even begin to develop these skills? The best way to start is by thinking about yourself: getting to understand yourself and how you relate to others. These are the first steps in developing what is known as 'emotional intelligence', which is a relatively recent leadership and management theory.

Emotional intelligence

There are numerous definitions of emotional intelligence (EI); mostly focusing on the importance of one's own feelings and emotions and how these affect not only your actions but the feelings and actions of those around you. This is what Stuart (2004) calls *emotional literacy*.

Leaders with EI are able to identify feelings and emotions in themselves and others and manage and reason with their emotions (Marquis and Huston, 2009). This sounds exceptionally challenging and there are ongoing debates in the literature as to whether EI is something that can be learned or whether it is an innate ability that some people possess and others do not. Salovey and Mayer (1990), recognised as the 'pioneers' of EI, suggested that EI is a skill that develops with age, that some people have a natural aptitude for and is therefore, difficult to learn. They refined their theory down to four specific mental abilities, or emotional building blocks of EI:

- The ability to actively perceive and express your own emotions
- The ability to integrate feelings and emotions into thought processes on demand, thereby facilitating an understanding of yourself and others
- The ability to understand emotions and what they mean for you and others
- The ability to regulate or manage your emotions.

(Vitello-Cicciu, 2003; Weisinger, 1998)

Conversely, Goleman (1998) argues that EI can actually be learned, although he agrees that it improves with age. He suggests that every person has a rational, thinking mind and an emotional, feeling mind, both of which influence how individuals act. Goleman (1998) identified five key elements of emotional intelligence, similar to those of Salovey and Mayer (1990):

Self-awareness – being able to recognise and understand your emotions, moods and drivers, as well as how these impact on others
Self-regulation – the ability to control any disruptive emotions or responses
Motivation – a drive to work towards a common goal
Empathy – being able to understand and accept other peoples' emotions, moods and drivers;
Social skills – the ability to build relationships and networks through finding common ground

(Goleman, 1998)

Applying Goleman's theories of EI to nursing, Reeves (2005) suggests that it is the self-regulation element of EI that allows nurses, regardless of their internal emotions, to work in a calm and professional manner during difficult or chaotic clinical situations. However, Goldman's theories of EI could equally be applied to Allied Health Professionals.

Weisinger (1998), agrees that EI can be learned, developed and directly applied to work situations. He suggests a six-step approach to developing your own emotional intelligence:

Developing high self-awareness – observing yourself in action and reflecting on what you see can help you to change and shape your actions appropriately

Managing your emotions – rather than suppressing your feelings and emotions, allowing yourself to feel and learning to understand and then manage your emotions can free you up to productively deal with difficult situations

Motivating yourself – having clarity about a task as well as drawing on external sources of support can help you to turn potential setbacks into positive outcomes

Developing effective communication skills – the wrong words or unclear messages can be damaging and so developing good, clear communication and listening skills are critical

Developing interpersonal expertise – being able to understand and analyse the many individual relationships you as a manager have to build and maintain is key. You are then able to communicate at the right levels at the right time with the right people

Helping others to help themselves – a successful team comprises more than one person and so helping others to manage their emotions, communicate effectively and become motivated is critical. Keeping your own emotional perspective and being a supportive listener can help others solve their problems and achieve their goals.

(Weisinger, 1998)

Most of the activities in the next section of this chapter are designed to help you to develop some of these key elements of EI.

Activities to enhance learning

This section contains some activities which will help you to think and reflect; not just on your skills and abilities as a manager but also about some of the factors that impact on how you might behave in certain situations. The activities will give you some insight into the decisions you make, why you make them and how you might think about your management practice in a different way, perhaps even changing what you do.

Activity 1: Reflective self assessment

For you to realise your full potential as a manager, it is essential for you to have a clear idea of your strengths and areas for development as well as having a reasonable idea of how others see you. This self-assessment activity will not give you all the answers but it will help; it will take a little time for you to complete but your patience and honesty will pay dividends and give you significant insights.

Have three short conversations, one with each of the following:

- Your manager
- Someone outside your organisation, like a peer or a mentor
- Yourself.

These are the sorts of questions you should ask yourself as well as your manager and peer:

- What are my strengths as a manager?
- Am I making the most of them now?
- Which strengths might be more valuable to me in the future?
- Which management skills or abilities do I need to develop?
- Is the lack of these skills holding me back at the moment? If so, why?
- Is it possible that not having these skills might hold me back in the future?
- How much do I really want to do something about them?
- What achievements am I most proud of this year?
- What things have motivated and enthused me this year as a manager?
- What experience have I gained this year?
- What have I learned from these positive experiences?
- What things have frustrated me this year? (These might be things like conflict, changes taking a long time to implement or things going badly).
- How did I respond to these at the time?
- What have I learned from these experiences?

continued . . .

Activity 1: Reflective self assessment ... *continued*

• What are the things I would really like to achieve as a manager in the short and long term?

Make a note of the answers; do they differ in any way? Do you see any patterns? What do the responses tell you about yourself as a manager? Do you think you are less capable than your manager thinks you are? Or are you more confident about your abilities than others around you think you are? What do you think you need to do to change the things you do least well?

Activity 2: What do I think is important as a manager?

It can be very helpful to identify what sort of manager you are by being clear about what you are *actually* focusing on in your work as a manager, rather than what you feel you *should* be achieving. It is natural for most managers to aim to facilitate their teams to achieve their overall objectives in a way which is efficient and effective, adhering to externally-set targets, within budget and in the meantime keeping your team happy and cohesive. However, this may not necessarily be what you are actually doing; these are inevitably competing interests and the nexus of all of these is where all managers wish to be, but rarely are.

Figure 5.1 shows a Venn diagram (Venn, 1880) of competing interests, showing each interest equally balanced with all the others, both in terms of size as well as overlap with each other. Achieving this is rare; in reality, most people move from focusing on different elements at different times depending on the situation as well as how they feel.

Draw your own competing interests diagram by thinking about the four areas listed below; try to be honest about what is most important to you most of the time. There are no right or wrong answers, just honest ones. Try to do this activity by thinking about what you actually feel and do, rather than what you feel you should be doing (i.e., having an equal set of circles!).

continued ...

Activity 2: What do I think is important as a manager?

. . . continued

Determine the size of each circle by how important you feel that aspect of your work is *to you*. You can do this by thinking about how much time and emotional energy you use in trying to achieve these outcomes. What makes you angry? What makes you happy? What makes you satisfied at the end of the day? Listening to your feelings can help you decide the size of each circle. Then decide which of the other areas that circle should overlap with and by how much. You may have additional competing interests that are not shown here which vie for your time and attention; ensure you add these: this is *your* diagram!

Reaching all targets – How important is ensuring that you meet all targets from within your own organisation as well as all government targets to you as a manager? How much time do you spend on making sure this happens and how much of the team's resources do you allocate to this? What prices are paid by you as an individual as well as by the team in the efforts to meet targets? (Reeves, 2005).

Maximising income and keeping within budgets – If you have the ability to increase income, how important is this to you and how much do you and your team focus on this element of the work? Do you like to keep within budget? Do you feel you will be harshly judged if you do not? Do you lose focus on other things in your attempts to maximise income and balance budgets?

Achieve all operational requirements – Do you focus on getting the job done, even if you do not always stay within budget and occasionally miss some targets? Is your focus the care of the patient and if it means going over budget a little, you feel able to justify this as you have done your job as a clinical team? What impact do you think this has on the team or the organisation as a whole?

Keeping the team happy and cohesive – Do you go out of your way to enable a close, effective and smooth-running team, who work well together? You may ensure you get things done in this way but you may sometimes go over-budget a little by e.g., getting holiday cover for the team or you may miss some targets, even though you feel these are important. Do you focus on the team because you want to be liked (Marquis and Huston, 2009), or because you feel a close team is an efficient one?

continued . . .

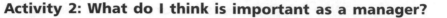

Activity 2: What do I think is important as a manager?

. . . continued

Being honest with yourself when doing this activity will help you to see what is actually important to you and will help you to identify areas to reflect on.

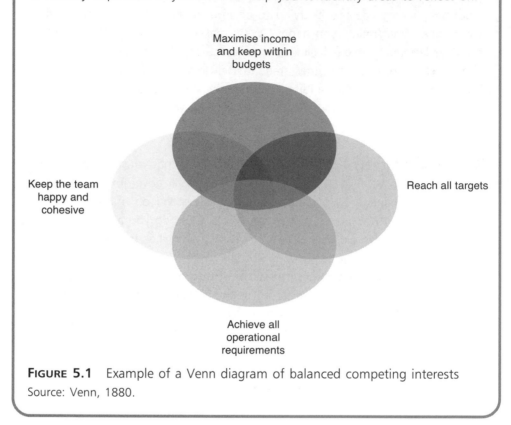

FIGURE 5.1 Example of a Venn diagram of balanced competing interests
Source: Venn, 1880.

Using a learning journal

We all have preferred ways of doing things in the workplace and as a manager. We may not realise it but we tend to do or respond to particular things in the same way most of the time; some people or situations just 'press our buttons' for some reason. It is entirely subconscious and instinctive. To develop as a manager one of the most powerful things we can do is to not only become *aware* of our 'buttons', our preferred ways of doing things, but to also gradually develop *choices* about how we do things or respond to situations: developing EI.

This is actually harder than it sounds; it means thinking critically and reflectively on things we have done or ways we have responded (Browne and Keeley, 2006). We may not always like what we see but this ability to reflect on situations helps us to get to know ourselves better and to spot the patterns and drivers to our responses. The aim is to see and understand your patterns *in the moment they occur* and then have choices about an appropriate response. Moving through these stages takes deep and honest reflection. A learning journal is a helpful tool you can use (Moon, 1999).

Try to keep your mind 'open' to significant events, interactions or triggers during your working day. Some of these might include times when you have had a strong feeling or response such as excitement, boredom, frustration, feeling frightened or feeling ignored. At some point in the day when something like this has occurred, make a little time to note the details briefly in a notebook. Come back to it later in the day or when you have a bit more time to complete the entry. You may simply be reflecting on your competing interests Venn diagram and finding that you have shifted your focus for some reason.

You may find that asking yourself the following questions helps you to focus on *you*: your role, responses and actions in any given situation. The questions can also be used to help you to structure your journal entries.

What was going on? Play the event back through your mind; try to remember what exactly happened, who said and did what, any key phrases said by you or others, what the body language of all the players was. This is not about recalling the outcome but rather the details of the entire event.

How was I feeling at the time? Try to recall what you were feeling while the event unfolded: Were you feeling anxious, excited, stressed, happy, and angry? Again, this is not always easy to do as we all have feelings we do not understand or acknowledge in ourselves. Being as honest as you can, when thinking about your feelings in a particular situation, will help you to see whether you respond in particular ways to certain feelings. Being aware of these automatic responses is the first step in changing those patterns.

What do I think this might mean? Can I make any connections here? Does this give me any insights into how I respond in particular situations or what my triggers are?

What can I try next time? How can I actively make the choice to respond in a different way when something like this happens again? Are there any strategies I could use which would make me act more consciously (i.e., counting to 10 before speaking or responding to a situation or waiting until the next day before responding to an email?).

Some tips on successful journal keeping

- Try to make a detailed, reflective entry in your journal around once a week if you can: it is not a diary so do not try to write something every day. Think of it as a process for you to use when there may be something for you to learn.
- Make the time to write your journal somewhere quiet when you will not be disturbed.
- Try to keep all your journal entries in one notebook, which is only used for that purpose.
- Once a month, go back and read through all the entries for that month in one go. Do you notice any patterns, any connections, and any particular triggers? If you do, what does this tell you about yourself? What have you learned about yourself? How might you do things differently next time? (Moon, 1999).

If you do manage to keep a regular learning journal and reflect on it on a monthly basis, you will find that you will be more aware of your feelings and responses and will start to 'be in the moment' much more. You will start responding in the way you would like to respond. You will also be much more aware of your own 'hooks' and 'traps': the people and situations which 'press your buttons' and to which you respond in a way that is emotional and raw rather than considered and of your choice.

Using reflective practice in meetings

We all have to attend meetings at times; some of us more than others. As a manager you may be responsible for chairing meetings and setting agendas. However, how many good and successful meetings can you truthfully say you have participated in? These were meetings in which everyone had their say; all matters on the agenda were appropriately dealt with in a timely fashion and clear decisions were made?

Certainly, one of the most satisfying moments at work is when you experience being part of a group working well together to solve a problem. Conversely, being part of a team which does not quite gel or does not get on top of a problem can be one of the most frustrating experiences at work. It is not uncommon to feel anxious about being excluded, blamed or insecure about our position in a meeting which is not well chaired. If you feel like this then it is likely that others may feel something similar, despite the Chair's best efforts to include everybody and cover the agenda comprehensively.

Think about effective meetings that you attend. What does the Chair do to make them effective? Looking at the following lists before and after a meeting (particularly if you are chairing) will help you to reflect more on your role in meetings, how you prepare for them and give you the tools to be an effective chair.

Things to think about before a meeting

- What is the purpose of the meeting?
- Are the right people invited? How well do they know each other?
- Does the agenda reflect the purpose of the meeting? Can anything be taken off? Does anything need to be added?
- Are there to be full minutes or just action points?
- Does any information need to be distributed in advance? If you want people to discuss and reach an agreement about, say, a lengthy policy, they need to see it ahead of the meeting.
- Who will lead each item on the agenda? It is a good idea to delegate agenda items to those best able to give the relevant information or lead the discussion. Agree in advance who will lead which discussion.
- Do the agenda items 'flow' well? It can be helpful to start with something easy and quick, with more difficult and long items in the middle and ending with shorter, 'clarifying things' items.
- Do not spend ages reviewing previous minutes: be familiar with the minutes and the agenda and be clear and concise about what is being carried forward onto the current agenda.
- How do you move between agenda items? Summarise the discussion and remind people of the decision.
- How do you keep to time? If a discussion has gone on longer than planned, consider suggesting coming back to the item next time; giving people a task to prepare for a decision at the next meeting. An example would be asking everyone to check what the preferences are within their team, or asking someone to get more information for next time.
- Be aware of shifts of energy as well as body language. Are people tired or bored? Can you bring that discussion to a prompt conclusion and move on to another agenda item?
- Be aware of your own feelings; others may be feeling the same.
- How do you end the meeting well? Quickly review the actions, decisions and next steps and thank people.
- Always finish on time!

Asking yourself the following questions *after* the meeting can also be helpful in giving you insight into the dynamics at the meeting as well as how you dealt with it.

- Who spoke most? Who spoke least? Why?
- Was the time spent on each agenda item used well? If not, how could that item have been dealt with more efficiently?
- Did people listen to each other and discuss matters openly?
- Which actions or people helped the meeting flow well?
- What actions or people do you think hindered the meeting's progress the most?

(Browne and Keeley, 2006)

Your responses to these questions and subsequent reflections will be telling and interesting. Consider trying something different at the next meeting: experiment with ideas and structures, or test your hypotheses by carefully looking to see if the same response occurs in a similar situation.

Reflecting on your power

There are many types of power that you, as an advanced level practice manager, have and use (Farrington, 2007). There are, however, numerous factors which may contribute to how much power you think you have as well as how much power other people *perceive* you to have. Some of these factors may seem obvious or trivial at first glance; some of them you will have control over while others are an innate part of you, or even a product of society's assumptions or expectations. Regardless, they are important for you to think about when trying to work out how others see you or experience your authority. Activity 3 can help you think about your power as a manager.

Activity 3

Look at the following list and think about what effect, if any, the factors below have on your power as a manager.

Gender – Are you 'given' more power because of your gender and if so, why? Do you 'take' more power because of your gender? Why? How does this interact with the gender of the people being managed?

continued . . .

Activity 3: ... *continued*

Nationality – Do you share the same nationality with some members of the team? What impact on your power does that have?

Educational background – Does having a similar social or educational background with some members of the team give you a special bond?

Looks – Does attractiveness give someone more or less power? Does wearing a suit (for men or women) mean that someone is given or takes more power?

Height – Can someone short have as much 'presence' as someone tall? If so, why?

History within the organisation – How important is it to have been working in the organisation for longer than others in the team? Or for significantly less time?

Experience – Does having more experience in your specialist area give you more power? Is it you who takes that power or others that give it to you?

(Adapted from Morgan, 1989; O'Regan and Ghobadian, 2004)

Understanding your power activity

Think about your current management role and functions on a daily basis and complete this over a period of one month. Come back to sections even when you think you have finished and will not make further changes or additions. Use the space to jot down your thoughts and any examples.

Use Table 5.1 overleaf to do this.

Case studies

Case studies are accepted as an innovative and thoughtful learning resource for managers in all fields of practice (Vitello-Cicciu, 2003; Mayo and Thompson, 1995; Salovey and Mayer, 1990). It is well documented that people can learn more effectively when actively involved in the learning process (Sivan et al., 2001; Bonwell and Eison, 1991). The case study approach is one way in which such active learning strategies can be implemented.

There are a number of definitions for the term 'case study'. For example, Fry et al. (1999) describe case studies as complex examples which give an

TABLE 5.1 Understanding your power activity

	How much of this power do I have? (None, some, a lot)	How often do I use this power? (Never, sometimes, often)
Positional or Legitimate Power Do you have formal authority in your role (i.e., take decisions or supervise other people)?		
Connection Power Are you close to someone who is powerful within the organisation and other people know you know them? Do you know powerful people outside the organisation?		
Resources Power Do you have control over resources: pay, promotion, training budgets, annual leave?		
Expert Power Do you have specialist knowledge or qualifications?		

(Adapted from Morgan, 1989)

insight into the context of a problem as well as illustrating the main point. In this chapter, a case study is defined as a person-centred activity based on topics that demonstrate theoretical concepts in an applied setting.

The following section has been compiled to help you to reflect on some of the more theoretical elements of this chapter as well as how you tackled and completed the practical activities. You will be able to apply some of the things you may have learned about yourself and about organisations to some practical scenarios.

Some of these scenarios position the participants in contexts which may be familiar to you. Even if you do not recall a similar incident, it is likely that you will have faced similar personal or professional dilemmas. By working through the case studies, you can reflect on what *you* would have done if you had been in that situation. This will help you to apply your knowledge of EI to resolve practical problems and issues and make thoughtful and appropriate decisions.

Case study 1

Josie is a newly appointed advanced practice clinical nurse manager in a long-established palliative care nursing team with a sound reputation in an inner city borough. Josie is new to the area and applied for the job as a sideways move, having already managed a similar but slightly smaller team in a different area. Part of the attraction of the job was how highly regarded the service is, as well as getting an opportunity to work with other experts in her chosen clinical field. The person who had previously held the management job had been in post for over five years and was an experienced manager and palliative care practitioner.

Josie's new team welcomed her warmly and were helpful and supportive in her first week. However, Josie felt anxious that she was somehow perceived as less experienced than her predecessor and in her first team meeting she felt insecure and shy when talking about her vision for the service. Her team were unclear about the changes that Josie was proposing and responded negatively, expressing their concerns for changing things that they perceived to be working well. As the meeting progressed, Josie felt more defensive and less certain about her proposals, and suggested that the team come back to the discussion after she had been able to get more information.

Josie wrote about the meeting in her learning journal and reflected on what had happened and how her feelings of inadequacy had led to her shyness and lack of confidence in the meeting. She reflected on whether she was indeed less experienced than her predecessor and was clear that she was as experienced, if not more so. For the next meeting, Josie prepared thoroughly, gathering data to support her proposals for change and approached the subject clearly and confidently. She used statements such as 'I think this is a good idea because . . .' and 'I think that our new rota will give patients an excellent service because . . .' The use of a personal statement such as 'I think . . .' helped Josie to clarify what she was thinking as well as recognising and reiterating that she is the person responsible for the service. By not saying that the new rota would provide *better* patient care, Josie reassured the team that she was not critical of the existing levels of patient care; reducing their negativity towards her. Her preparation and confidence in presenting her vision for the service further inspired her team to get behind the proposed changes.

Case study 2

Paul shares a caseload with his colleague, Sam, but they work in different offices on the same floor and often have to use the same files, just at different times. Paul feels that he is careful to ensure that he always returns the files after he has used them but finds that Sam hangs onto files on his desk, meaning that Paul spends time looking for them in the drawer and then has to go and look on Sam's desk or ask for them when he needs them. Despite Paul's regular requests to Sam to put the files back in the drawer once he has finished with them, Sam continues to hold onto files regularly. Paul feels angry, disrespected and that Sam never listens to him. Every time he looks for a file and cannot find it he feels angry. It is affecting how he responds to Sam at other times.

Sam does not understand why Paul is so grumpy in the office all the time and assumes that Paul does not like him. He also begins to wonder if Paul's grumpiness is because he is getting burnt out clinically, but decides to keep an eye on things and not discuss his concerns with a manager yet.

Paul attends a course where he is encouraged to keep a reflective journal. After a month of entries, Paul reads his journal and notes that he has been writing as much on his anger towards Sam as on the care of the patients on his caseload. Paul decides he must take some action and starts to pay close attention to how he responds each time he finds that Sam has not returned a file to the drawer. He realises that once he has one negative thought about Sam, such as 'why doesn't he listen to me?', a 'domino effect' of feelings follows. He finds himself thinking further negative thoughts towards Sam such as 'what is wrong with him?', 'he is so selfish' or 'I wish he would just leave'.

Paul realised that he was generalising about Sam and making wild interpretations of Sam's behaviour. He thought carefully and realised that

Sam is actually not selfish in other ways and he certainly listens to Paul and respects his opinion when they discuss patients or other matters. He decides to tell Sam how upsetting he finds not being able to find files when he needs them. Paul talks about how hard he finds the situation, and how frustrating and time-consuming it is and asks Sam if there is some way they can resolve the matter. Paul even suggests that he would be happy to come and get the files from Sam's office once he has finished with them if he lets Paul know when he is done with them.

Sam is astonished that Paul feels so strongly about the files and is immensely relieved that a simple solution can be found to his absent-mindedness. Understanding how upsetting Paul finds not being able to find shared files makes Sam more conscious of what he does with files when he has finished with them and over a short period of time, their working relationship improves hugely.

Conclusion

In this chapter we have learned how important it is to have a sound awareness of our own feelings and how these can impact on our behaviour, as well as that of others. Keeping a learning journal for reflection can be a valuable tool and doing this regularly over a minimum of one year can help us to identify any patterns in our feelings or behaviour in particular situations. Although there is no magic formula for becoming the perfect manager, these final key reminders might be helpful:

- Step back and notice what is happening around you: reflect on the dynamics of every interaction you are part of before speaking or acting
- There is no need to have a personality transplant: know your strengths and weaknesses, reflect on these and work to change your responses
- Get help with reflection: get a mentor, join a peer support group and keep a reflective diary
- If something is not working, try a new strategy
- Your management style may need to differ and adapt according to the person or situation
- Being a good listener makes you a better advanced level practice manager.

References

Bonwell, C. C. and Eison, J. A. (1991) *Active Learning: Creating Excitement in the Classroom.* ASHE-ERIC Higher Education Report No. 1. Washington, DC: The George Washington University, School of Education and Human Development.

Browne, M. and Keeley, S. M. (2006) (Eds). *Asking the right Questions: a guide to critical thinking.* (8th edition). New Jersey: Prentice Hall.

Department of Health and Social Security (1983) *The NHS Management Enquiry. Griffiths Report.* London: HMSO.

Department of Health (1998). *A First Class Service: Quality in the New NHS.* London: HMSO.

—— (2000) *The NHS Plan.* London: HMSO.

Farrington, J. (2007) *Top 7 Sources of Personal Power.* Available from: http://Top7Business.com/?expert=Jonathan_Farrington (accessed 14/06/2011)

Fry, H., Ketteridge, S. and Marshall, S. (1999) *A Handbook for Teaching and Learning in Higher Education.* Glasgow: Kogan Page.

Goleman, D. (1998) *Working with Emotional Intelligence.* New York: Bantam Books.

Iles, V. and Sutherland, K. (2002) *Organisational Change: A Review for Healthcare Managers, Professionals and Researchers.* London: NIHR Service Delivery and Organisation Programme. Available from: http://www.sdo.nihr.ac.uk/managingchange.html (accessed 14/06/2011)

Marquis, B. L. and Huston, C. J. (2009) *Leadership Roles and Management functions in Nursing: theory and application* (6th Ed). London: Wolters Kluwer Health/Lippincott Williams and Wilkins.

Marsaili, C., Cranfield, S., Iles, V. and Stone, J. (2001) *Managing Change in the NHS: Making Informed Decisions on Change.* London: NHS Service Delivery and Organisation at London School of Hygiene and Tropical Medicine. Available from: http://www.sdo.nihr.ac.uk/files/adhoc/change-management-booklet.pdf (accessed 14/06/2011)

Mayo, M. and Thompson, J. (1995) *Adult Learning: Critical Intelligence and Social Change.* London: National Institute of Adult Continuing Education.

Moon, J. (1999) *Learning Journals: A Handbook for Academics, Students and Professional Development.* London: Kogan Page.

Morgan, G. (1989) *Images of Organisations.* London: Sage.

O'Regan, N. and Ghobadian, A. (2004) Leadership and Strategy: making it happen. J*ournal of General Management*, 29(3): 76–92.

Reeves, A. (2005) Emotional Intelligence. *American Association of Occupational Health Nurses Journal*, 53(4): 172–76.

Salovey, P. and Mayer, J. D. (1990) Emotional Intelligence. *Imagination, cognition and personality*, 9(1990): 185–211.

Salter, B. (2004) *The New Politics of Medicine.* Basingstoke: Palgrave Macmillan.

Sivan, A., Wong, L. R., Woon, C. and Kember, D. (2001) An Implementation of Active Learning and its Effect on the Quality of Student Learning. *Innovations in Education and Training International*, 37(4): 381–89.

Stuart, P. (2004) Emotional Intelligence: developing emotionally literate training in mental health. *Mental Health Practice*, 8(4): 12–15.

Venn, J. (1880) On the diagrammatic and mechanical representation of propositions and reasonings. *Philosophical Magazine and Journal of Science*, 9(59): 1–18.

Vitello-Cicciu, J. M. (2003) Exploring Emotional intelligence. *Journal of Nursing Administration*, 33(4): 203–10.

Weisinger, H. (1998) *Emotional Intelligence at Work.* San Francisco: Jossey Bass.

Chapter 6 Advanced Nursing Practice in the United States of America: Managing, negotiating and monitoring the healthcare system

Jane Sumner

Introduction

This chapter will enable you to critically discuss and explore the role of the advanced practice nurse (APN) in healthcare delivery in the United States of America (USA), the different specialties of advanced practice nursing, and the various organisations that influence/control it. Advanced nursing education is included, as is practice with all the issues the nurse must consider and attend to as he/she negotiates a fraught professional landscape. To negotiate the system, nurses need to be cognisant of major issues that relate to licensure, accreditation, certification and education (LACE) for advanced practice because they influence where nurses will practice and how they will practice. Barriers to practice that relate to advanced nursing practice satisfaction are also discussed.

Learning outcomes

At the conclusion of this chapter you will be able to:

- Explicate the multiple pressures influencing advanced practice nursing in the USA
- Examine the different licensing, accreditation, certification and educational issues associated with APN practice in the USA
- Understand issues related to negotiating and managing practice as an APN.

Background

In the United States of America (USA) the population is ageing and unlike the United Kingdom (UK), in which healthcare is provided free via the National Health Service (NHS), fewer Americans have healthcare insurance coverage which limits access to service. Chronic disease management is becoming more problematic with increasing obesity and its attendant illnesses e.g., diabetes mellitus, hypertension, and cardiovascular disease. However, Healthcare Reform became federal law as the *Patient Health Protection and Affordable Care Law* and the *Health Care and Education Reconciliation Practice Act* in March 2010. This will change how healthcare is delivered (Public Health Law 111–148, 2011). This law will force a paradigmatic shift from episodic, acute illness care to health promotion, wellness, disease prevention and optimal management of chronic disease. It opens up opportunities for APNs as never before – providing they are willing to take advantage of the change. The ongoing shift is inexorably towards primary care in neighbourhood clinics, and a 'medical home' for every American citizen. APNs who have specialised in geriatrics, family, adult, paediatrics, and women's health are well positioned for practice in the delivery model.

The shift to primary care raises concerns because of the ongoing and projected shortage of primary care doctors. In 2008, only 2% of all new doctors selected primary care as their specialty (Hauer et al., 2008). Unfortunately, by 2030, 20% of the American population will be more than 65 years old (He et al., 2005) and historically it is the older population that has greater need of healthcare services. APNs are increasingly 'filling this gap while maintaining quality care and often lowering health care costs' (Stanley et al., 2009:341), and presumably continue to do so.

One study by Brooten et al. (2003) studied five groups of patient problems and the difference APNs made in terms of improving patient outcomes. The most important function of the APN was surveillance of physiological and psychosocial needs, and the patient's environment: followed by health teaching; guidance and counselling; case management and finally treatments and procedures. These functions reduced hospital length of stay and home visits assisted in preventing readmissions for considerable cost savings. What this suggests is that the APN is providing quality primary health care with excellent patient outcomes; cost effectively. As Stanley et al. (2009) state:

> 'Nurses are arguably in the best position to realize the goals of health care reform, which include enhancing access to affordable care, providing patient-centered care, focusing on wellness and prevention, improving

quality and outcomes of care, emphasizing chronic illness management, assisting patients in making informed choices, and improving care coordination.'

(Stanley et al., 2009:340).

Advanced practice nursing

APNs in the USA are registered nurses who have received masters-level (graduate) education, which is built on baccalaureate education and practice. There are many specialties to select from, and, like in the UK, APNs may practice independently or in an interprofessional team, in acute care or non acute care. Within acute care, APNs may practice in specialised units e.g., in different intensive care units, the emergency room, or specialty outpatient clinics (i.e., pain management or diabetes management). In the non-acute environment APNs may practice in long term care, specialty rehabilitation facilities, community health/neighbourhood health clinics, public health/ community health, schools, prisons, retail-based clinics, or occupational health.

Many Registered Nurses (RNs) in the USA, as in the UK, select the graduate education that builds on their practice experience (i.e., the nurse who works in a neonatal intensive care unit may well decide to become a neonatal nurse practitioner). Others will opt for something quite different i.e., the nurse who has run a large outpatient clinic may choose to become a public health/ community health nurse. In the USA, those nurses who decide they want to become a Certified Registered Nurse Anaesthetist (CRNA) are required to have practiced in a surgical intensive care unit for a designated period of time before being admitted to that specialty educational programme, and are certificated in Advanced Cardiac Life Support (ACLS).

The APN is an independent, autonomous practitioner, practicing under his/her own license. The acronyms APN and APRN (i.e., Advanced Practice Registered Nurse) are equally accepted by the State Boards of Nursing (Easom, 2005) as descriptors of nurses who have received nursing education and have acquired certification and/or licensure as an advanced practice nurse (APRN, 2008). There are, however, many different types of, or titles for APNs to further confuse the issue: Clinical Nurse Specialist (CNS); Clinical Nurse Leader (CNL), this nurse is regarded as a generalist practicing at an advanced level and who remains in acute hospital practice; Advanced Practice Registered Nurse (APRN); Nurse Practitioner (NP); Certified Registered Nurse Anaesthetist (CRNA); Certified Nurse Midwife (CNM); and more recently the Doctor of Nursing Practice (DNP). Within the 'nurse practitioner' nomenclature, there are further subspecialties i.e., Family Nurse Practitioner

(FNP) or Geriatric Nurse Practitioner (GNP). In addition the APN may become certified in any one of number of specialties that do not have required specialist licensure i.e., enterostomal nursing or oncology or palliative care nursing.

Some of these specialties will be eligible for prescriptive authority e.g., NP, or not e.g., CNS. Each of the 50 states and the District of Columbia allow for some form of prescriptive authority. In some states APNs have limited prescriptive authority, usually within some sort of organisational protocols, similar to the Patient Group Directions (PGDs) used in many NHS Trusts in the UK. Other states permit unfettered prescriptive authority, and still other states will allow unfettered prescriptive authority except for the ordering of narcotics. Prescriptive authority covers not only the ordering of medications, but also the ordering of laboratory tests and durable medical equipment. Some APNs will indeed practice truly autonomously and independently, but others will practice under a doctor or in collaboration with one. Some APNs will practice in acute hospital care and others will practice in non-acute care sites. The expectation of the APN regardless of title and education is to: be a leader of the interprofessional team; enable nurse colleagues to utilise evidence-based practice principles; communicate effectively with all members of the team including patient and family (Tuite and George, 2010). Studies reveal that most patients in the USA are satisfied with the care received from APNs and in some instances more than satisfied with that care than that received from doctors or physician assistants (Agosta, 2009), or mainly because of their holistic approach to both patient and family particularly in shared medical appointments (Watts, et al., 2009) which is a similar finding in the UK (Cox et al., 2010; Cox and Hall, 2007).

Activity 1

Consider the Introduction Chapter in this book. Issues were raised regarding the variety of titles associated with the APN role. Issues were also raised regarding regulation (licensure) of practice. What issues do you see in relation to the aforementioned? Are there lessons that can be learned from the USA?

Licensure, Accreditation, Certification and Education (LACE)

Understanding advanced nursing practice in the USA has become increasingly complex, partly because of the different organisations weighing in on different aspects of it: whether it is legislative or regulatory, this latter includes 'educators, certifiers, and licensing bodies' (Stanley et al., 2009:341). These organisations include the American Association of Colleges of Nursing (AACN) (AACN, 2009) and the National League for Nursing (NLN), which accredit schools of nursing; specialist certification bodies e.g., American Nurses Credentialing Center (ANCC); the licensure organisation, the National Council of State Boards of Nursing (NCSBN) with individual state boards; the National Association of Clinical Nurse Specialists (NACNS) which has identified core competencies required of all CNS's and is developing core education requirements, and finally, different specialty organisations which have their own scope and standards of practice e.g., the National Organisation of Nurse Practitioner Faculties (NONPF), or the American Academy of Nurse Practitioners (AANP), or the Council of Anesthesia (COA).

A number of recent reports from the Institute of Medicine (IOM) (To Err is Human, 1999; Crossing the Quality Chasm, 2001; Priority Areas for National Action: Transforming Healthcare Quality, 2003a; Future of the Public's Health in the 21st Century, 2003b; Who will Keep the Public Healthy, 2003c) make clear that the USA cannot continue with its highly dysfunctional healthcare delivery system, which is fragmentary at best, very expensive, and has some of the worst health indices of the developed world. These reports reveal concerns about access to healthcare services, the quality of the services provided, and what needs to be done to improve them. Five core competencies have been recommended to be included in the education of all healthcare professionals (HCPs) and to be implemented in practice:

- Provide patient-centred care
- Work in interdisciplinary teams
- Employ evidence-based practice
- Apply quality improvement
- Utilize informatics.

(Finkelman and Kenner, 2007)

Partly, but not only because of these reports, 44 national nursing organisations came together to reach a consensus on what APRN regulation should be. A working group was formed that produced the Consensus Document, which is supported by the NCSBN, and has become the standard for LACE. There were four goals established by the working group:

- To strive for harmony and common understanding in the APRN community to promote quality APRN education and practice

- To develop an agreed-to vision for APRN regulation, including education, accreditation, certification, and licensure
- To establish a set of standards that protect the public, improve mobility, and improve access to safe, quality APRN care
- To produce a written framework that reflects consensus on APRN regulatory issues and strengthens the APRN position within the health care system.

(Stanley et al., 2009:344)

Within the Consensus Document, the APRN roles have been identified as Nurse Anaesthesia, Nurse Midwife, Clinical Nurse Specialist, and Nurse Practitioner. The population foci are: family/individual across the lifespan, adult gerontology, neonatal, paediatrics, women's health/gender related, and psychiatric mental health. Other specializations i.e., oncology or palliative care, or orthopaedics are also included in APRN practice, providing the nurse has received graduate education in the specialty. What is not specifically included in the Consensus Document is that nursing administration and public health/community health nursing are not regarded as APRN practice specialties. However as Stanley et al. (2009) attest, the Consensus Document has not yet been fully implemented and its success ultimately is contingent on national acceptance and implementation. This seems to suggest that there may still be room for negotiation, but that is by no means clear. The concerns for those in nursing administration and public health nursing rest on the issue of advanced courses in health assessment, pathophysiology and pharmacy (3Ps) that are necessary knowledge for APRNs, but which are not curricula content or necessary for practice in these two specialties.

Not only does AACN accredit schools of nursing, within its arm the Crediting Commission Nursing Education (CCNE), but so does the National League of Nursing within its National League for Nursing Accrediting Commission (NLNAC). It seems however that the AACN Essentials document has had a greater influence on graduate nursing education than the NLNAC and therefore it is the model utilized most frequently. From an educational perspective the AACN has mandated the Essentials of Master's Nursing Education, which provides the required curricula content and also the framework of a school's organisational structure. Meeting the Essentials is required of schools accredited by CCNE (Refer to Table 6.1).

The Consensus Document has already been adopted by the National Association of Clinical Nurse Specialists (NACNS), as it developed core educational competencies required for CNSs. These educational competencies have been derived from the Three Spheres of Influence in Patient Care: Patient/Client

TABLE 6.1 Essentials of Master's Nursing Education

Essential I	Scientific Underpinnings for Practice
Essential II	Organisational & Systems Leadership
Essential III	Quality Improvement & Safety
Essential IV	Translational Scholarship for Evidence-Based Practice and Innovation
Essential V	Information Systems/Technology & Patient Care for the Improvement of Health Care
Essential VI	Health Policy & Advocacy
Essential VII	Inter-professional Collaboration for Improving Patient and Population Health Outcomes
Essential VIII	Clinical Prevention & Population Health for Improving Health
Essential IX	Master's-Level Nursing Practice (Advancing Professionalism & Professional Values)

American Association of Colleges of Nursing Master's Essentials (2011)

Sphere; the Nurses/Nursing Sphere; and the System/Organisational Sphere (Goudreau et al., 2007:311) that constitute practice competencies domains. They stated that 'clinical expertise in a specialty is the hallmark of CNS practice ... [having] clinical expertise in diagnosis and treatment used to prevent, remediate or alleviate illness and promote health within a defined specialty population.' (Goudreau et al., 2007:311).

State boards of nursing

The power of the state boards of nursing (BON) should never be under-estimated because of their policing responsibility to keep the public safe. Each of the BONs in the 50 states and the District of Columbia have regulatory control, which means these organisations have final responsibility for controlling practice authority, reimbursement and prescriptive authority. Each BON has its own Practice Act, which has been passed by its State Legislature and is periodically reopened for necessary and timely changes. Each BON is made up of nurses from different aspects of the profession e.g., practice and education. The governor of a state makes the final selection of BON members and in many states a term lasts for four years. The BON meets monthly to discuss issues of concern that relate to policing and regulation. This body has the responsibility of licensing nurses but also of removing nurse's licenses for egregious actions (similar to the Nursing and Midwifery Council [NMC] in the UK). In the case of (suspected) egregious actions, the nurse is given a fair hearing to ensure that all the evidence is taken into account before a punishment (if required) is decided. Thus the ultimate autonomy of the APN rests with the BONs that decide the professional's ability to be able to make decisions within the limits of the education, skill, and professional competency of the provider which results in efficient use of resources (BHPR, 2010).

In 1973, Idaho became the first state to pass legislation granting APNs 'supervisory, collaborative, and independent authority to practice' (Phillips, 2010:24). Since then every state has followed suit although the degree of responsibility and autonomy varies from state to state. There is no federal right of control over state rights in this instance. It is the state that grants licensure and prescriptive authority to the individual ANP. This means that as an ANP moves from state to state he or she must be cognisant of the rules and regulations for practice of the state in which he or she is practicing.

Scope and standards of practice

The scope and standards of practice of many different specialties, at both general and specialist levels have been published by the American Nurses Association (ANA) as well as many specialty organizations. These essentially define the competencies expected of all APNs, as well the limits of a specialty practice (ANA, 2007). The role of Advanced Nurse Practitioners defined by the Scope and Standards of Nurse Practitioners (AANP, 2002), as 'they . . . are primary care providers . . . Nurse practitioners practice autonomously and in collaboration with health care professionals and other individuals to diagnose, treat and manage the patient's health problems' (American Academy of Nurse Practitioners 2002b cited by Weilland, 2008:347). Refer to Table 6.2 for the Domains and competencies for Nurse Practitioners (NPs) that have been produced by the National Organisation of Nurse Practitioner Faculties (NONPF, 2006). These Domains and competencies correspond with the Domains and competencies produced by the NMC (2005) and the Royal College of Nursing (RCN, 2008).

According to Stewart et al. (2010), the American Academy of Nurse Practitioners in its 2007 *Standards of Practice* document outlined 'qualifications, process of care, care priorities, collaborative responsibilities, documentation requirements, patient advocacy responsibilities, quality assurance, adjunct roles, and research initiatives' (Stewart et al., 2010:27) for all NPs. The emphasis is on NP responsibility, comprehensive assessment and decision making.

Individual nurse practice within a specialty can be evaluated according to the specific standards regardless of which organisation provides them

TABLE 6.2 Domains and core competencies of NPs

Domains	Core Competencies
One	Management of Patient Health/Illness Status
Two	The Nurse–Practitioner–Patient Relationship
Three	The Teaching–Coaching Function
Four	A Professional Role
Five	Managing and Negotiating Health Care Delivery Systems
Six	Monitoring and Ensuring the Quality of HealthCare Practice
Seven	Culturally Sensitive Care

National Organisation of Nurse Practitioner Faculties Domains and Core Competencies of Nurse Practitioner Practice (2006).

(i.e., COA, NONPF or ANA). The ANA's Public Health Nursing Scope and Standards of Practice are provided in Table 6.3 as an example of specific specialty standards.

Master's Preparation or Doctor of Nursing Practice

Unfortunately, the nurse who is seeking advanced practice has many issues to confront when selecting an education programme which will drive future practice. No longer are the choices limited to a Master's degree, largely because of the number of clinical practicum hours required of NP and CRNA education; thus increasing the total number of credit hours required for graduation. The AACN proposed that a Doctor of Nursing Practice (DNP) degree should be the degree of choice particularly for the two specialties mentioned. The AACN is calling for all schools that offer these two specialties to provide a DNP by 2015. However AACN is not limiting this degree to only CRNAs and NPs. Rather it indicates that there are two different patient care foci for this degree: direct patient care which requires all of these APNs to have completed the 3Ps, and indirect patient care which does not require the 3Ps; so all specialties are included. This means that both nursing administration and public health/community health nursing will also be included in DNP degrees.

There have been a number of arguments posited on why the nursing profession needs to have a DNP. One of the leading reasons has been to achieve parity with other health care professions i.e., pharmacy, physical therapy, occupational therapy and audiology. Another reason is how advanced education improves patient outcomes. The number of credit hours required

TABLE 6.3 ANA's Public Health Nursing Scope and Standards of Practice

Public Health Nursing Competencies	Scope and Standards of Public Health Nursing Practice	Standards of Practice for Public Health Nursing
Proficiency: Advanced Mastery of the competency. Individuals are able to synthesize, critique or teach the skill	Tenets	Standard 1: Assessment
		Standard 2: Population Diagnosis and Priorities
Domain 1	1. Population-based assessment, policy development, and assurance processes are systematic and comprehensive	Standard 3: Outcomes Identification
Analytic Assessment Skills		Standard 4: Planning
Domain 2		Standard 5: Implementation
Policy Development/Programme Planning Skills	2. All processes must include partnering with representatives of the people	Standard 5A: Coordination of Services
		Standard 5B: Heath Education and Health Promotion
Domain 3	3. Primary prevention is given priority	Standard 5C: Consultation
Communication Skills	4. Intervention strategies are selected to create healthy environmental, social, and economic conditions in which people can thrive	Standard 5D: Regulatory Activities
Domain 4		Standard 6: Evaluation
Cultural Competency Skills		Standards of Professional Performance
Domain 5	5. Public health nursing practice includes an obligation to actively reach out to all who might benefit from an intervention	Standard 7: Quality of Care
Community Dimensions of Practice Skills		Standard 8: Education
		Standard 9: Professional Practice Evaluation
Domain 6	6. The dominant concern and obligation is for the greater good of all of the people or population as a whole	Standard 10: Collegiality and Professional Relationships
Basic Public Health Sciences Skills		
Domain 7		Standard 11: Collaboration
Financial Planning and Management Skills		Standard 12: Ethics
	7. Stewardship and allocation of available resources supports the maximum population health benefit gain	Standard 13: Research
Domain 8		Standard 14: Resource Utilisation
Leadership and Systems Thinking Skills		Standard 15: Leadership
	8. The health of the people is most effectively promoted and protected through collaboration with members of other professions and organisations	Standard 16: Advocacy

ANA (2007)

122

in certain specialties to achieve this, e.g., CRNA, is more than required for a regular Master's degree. Furthermore, the salary has the potential to be higher. Upvall and Ptachcinski (2007) compared nursing with pharmacy. They discovered that nursing initially led the way towards this advanced degree but it was pharmacy who in fact introduced a professional doctorate before nursing. The primary rationales for a PharmD degree were a 'societal healthcare need that occurred as pharmacotherapy became an increasingly important component' (Upvall and Ptachcinski, 2007:317) and the increasing knowledge of pharmacology, pharmacokinetics and clinical pharmacotherapy. Similar rationales can be provided for nursing and pharmacy has provided nursing with the necessary direction.

Although AACN has mandated the DNP in lieu of the traditional Master's degree by 2015, there is debate on the wisdom of this and whether some specialties would be better served by only offering a Master's degree or perhaps both degrees. Avery and Howe (2007) discuss the pros and cons of a Master's in Nurse-Midwifery versus a DNP as a result of a survey of 110 certified nurse midwives (CNM). The results revealed that although the Directors of Midwifery Education have endorsed AACN with a position statement (that has a number of caveats) there seems to be no resolution on the appropriate course of action, and there are insufficient data to date to support a DNP. Because a DNP would take longer than a traditional Master's degree issues related to increased cost were raised, and whether as many nurses would apply for a DNP in Nurse-Midwifery, which would further increase the shortage of CNMs. More practicum hours would be required, and this could further stress what is already a difficulty in finding enough clinical sites and appropriately prepared preceptors. However 68 of the surveyed nurses did indicate that they believed a DNP would increase their stature. Present DNP programmes already address AACN's Eight Essentials. Whether to move from a Master's degree to a DNP further confounds the problem for this specialty because not all midwives are nurse-midwives. They are certified midwives who have not completed the nursing component in a school of nursing.

This chapter reveals some under-discussed issues as schools moving from the traditional Master's programmes, be they CNS or APRN to the DNP. Length of education and cost are serious considerations, and upon graduation whether there will be jobs available with commensurate salaries. For associate degree prepared nurses (ADN) who aim for graduate education these problems are even greater as they have to move through the different educational levels (Bachelor of Science Degree [BSc]; Master of Science [MSc]).

Activity 2

Reflect on your present level of education and training. Is it essential for you to obtain additional education and training to achieve your goal of becoming an ANP? If 'yes', at what level should your education and training be directed?

Identify the current pros and cons to obtaining an ANP qualification. Are you in a position to take action now? If 'yes' what initiatives are required for you to take action?

If you are presently practicing as an ANP, what level of education and training do you have? Is it sufficient to maintain your position as an ANP? If 'no' what additional education and training do you think is required?

Practice issues

The nurse, having made the decision on a specialty practice and an educational programme, has more issues to confront on graduation. He or she must consider where he/she wants to practice and whether or not prescriptive authority is something he/she believes he/she must have, and he/she must find the information to ensure the right decision is made. Once educated and licensed as an APN, then where to practice becomes the central issue. Furthermore, the APN will have to confront barriers that confound that practice. This is more so in the very fluid healthcare delivery world, which is currently the USA system, as healthcare reform goes from enacted law into policy, rules and regulations. If the new APN is going to practice within a collaborative doctor practice, then should that APN charge under his/her own license and credentials, or should he/she bill under the collaborating doctor's name?

Regardless of the changes that are coming, at the present time the newly minted APN in the USA is required to take the specialty certification examination; apply for state licensure; consider how he/she will achieve the continuing education credits for re-licensure; take out malpractice insurance; ensure the number of annual practice hours that are required for ongoing certification; understand billing and reimbursement issues, along with the different reimbursement mechanisms depending on who the third-party payer is; and if planning to open an independent business then develop a business plan and ensure that it is not undercapitalised, if it is going to be sustained.

For those APNs who are going to practice within facilities that are accredited by Joint Commission (which accredits acute care facilities and many non-acute care facilities i.e., home health agencies in the USA), then they will have to undertake the process of credentialing and privileging. Credentialing refers to the 'process of verifying education, licensure, and certification to practice as an advanced practice nurse, whereas privileging involves granting the authority to perform specific aspects of patient care' (Kleinpell et al., 2008:279). Scope of practice is underscored by the process of credentialing and privileging, and ensures that the nurse meets the standards of the specialty of the position sought, and that the nurse is indeed educated, licensed and certificated for that particular position; if not then the APN is unable to work in that position. Credentialing and privileging 'promote[s] accountability, enforce[s] professional standards of practice, enable[s] third party billing for services, and communicate[s] the scope of practice to other professionals' (Kleinpell et al., 2008:279). Increasingly the potential employer will require a criminal record check (CRB) of the candidate and can request the [federal] National Practitioner Data Bank provide information regarding 'licensure disciplinary actions, malpractice payments or adverse actions affecting professional memberships' (Kleinpell et al., 2008:280). According to Joint Commission accreditation requirement the APN must be evaluated regularly with reappointment two to three years post-hire if appropriate. The six competencies now required by Joint Commission in relation to medical staff, and which APNs must now meet are: 'patient care skills; medical knowledge, interpersonal and communication skills, professionalism, practice-based learning and systems-based practice' (Kleinpell et al., 2008:286).

For some APNs a Convenient Care Clinic (CCC) may be the practice site of choice in partnership with other APNs. These clinics are not uncommonly located in shopping malls, and treat minor acute illnesses 'such as sore throats, upper respiratory infections, fevers, rashes and urinary tract infections' (Evans, 2010:24), but no chronic illnesses, with flexible hours 24 hours a day 7 days a week. Evans stated that these clinics 'offer convenience, value, location, quality and cost' (Evans, 2010:24), and reduce pressures on over-crowded emergency rooms (accident and emergency departments) and urgent care clinics. All patients are charged small, cash only rates which are posted outside the clinic, no credit cards accepted – which is important for those patients with no health insurance. Some APNs prefer rural practice rather than urban practice, and indeed they may be the only healthcare providers in many underserved rural states.

One small, convenience sample study completed in the north eastern USA demonstrates the practice of NPs in a variety of non-institutional settings.

Deshefy-Longhi et al. (2008) present results from electronic data collection of the 54 NPs who chose to participate. These nurses were practicing in paediatric, family, adult, women's health and geriatric practice: most of which were home visits to the elderly in assisted living facilities; in private paediatric and obstetric clinics; and in community based clinics. Most of the visits by patients were for acute health problems, with 'only 30% of visits for chronic illness management (either routine care or treatment of an exacerbation) and even fewer for health promotion' (Deshefy-Longhi et al., 2008:286), but the NPs did provide routine screenings and annual checkups. However, the NPs offered health promotion and disease prevention teaching and counselling; particularly in comparison with doctors who participated in similar electronic data collection studies. Interestingly, these nurses prescribed medication in 63% of cases for the acute problem visit and for the primary diagnosis. Anything more specific would depend on the NP's specialty and his/her patient population (i.e., the paediatric population would be different and have different needs from the geriatric population). 40% of reimbursement came from Medicaid, self pay (because of no healthcare insurance) or no pay, suggesting the bulk of these nurses' patients were poor and/or minority patients. The limitation of this study is the small sample and the patient populations seen. However it does provide an indication of a typical NP non-institutional practice (Deshefy-Longhi et al., 2008).

Third party payers and reimbursement

Obviously the APN expects to be paid for services rendered but how this is set up depends on the state, the type of practice and the type of specialty. In the USA there are two 'public' sources of funding for healthcare services.

The federal government funds Medicare which is medical insurance available for those over the age of 65 years. It is complicated by the fact that different parts pay for different services: Part A pays for hospital services for when a person is an inpatient, and Part B pays for doctor services on an outpatient basis. The latter requires significant monthly co-pay. Part C is a combination of both Medicare Parts A & B generally offered at a lower cost to the original Medicare, but is administered by private insurance companies who put the patient into a network with specific doctors and hospitals, which may limit services. Part D is the medication coverage component, but this has limits in coverage. Medicare only reimburses for 80% of the cost of services provided. This means that those who can afford it will have ongoing private insurance which will pay 80% of the outstanding 20% of the bill. Patients are required to pay some sort of co-pay, and this can be variable. Under the 1997 Federal

Balanced Budget Act Medicare was authorized to reimburse APRNs (including NPs, CNSs and CRNAs) at all practice sites, but at rates that were only 85% of doctor rates (Mercer Ray, 2008).

Medicaid, which largely provides care for the indigent, is a state run health care financing organisation that decides what service in a particular state will be covered (i.e., how much is reimbursed for home care, how much is reimbursed for days in an acute care hospital, how much to reimburse doctors, but is supported with both federal [the majority amount] and state funding). Many APNs are reimbursed under Medicaid, but if in solo practice may or may not be reimbursed under Medicare. In some Medicaid state programmes the APN is reimbursed for services at 100% of the doctor fee, and in other states the APN is reimbursed at only 70% or 80% of doctor fees.

Similar to Medicaid is a programme of medical insurance specifically for children called the State Children's Health Insurance Programme (SCHIP) which is a combination of both federal and state monies. This means that all children without healthcare insurance have access to services including routine vaccinations and checkups.

One other federal programme that both provides services and pays for them is the Veterans Health Administration (VHA), which is available nationwide. Services covered include in hospital care, rehabilitation, nursing home, home health, doctor and APN services, and some medication assistance. Veterans of wars with no other health insurance are eligible for services, and in some instances so are their families. Those who return wounded from on-going wars are not initially included in the VHA, but once they are discharged from military hospital services they are. Studies demonstrate that VHA patients are satisfied with APN services and job satisfaction amongst these nurses is high as well (Faris, et al., 2010; Watts et al., 2009). In fact Watts et al. (2009) stated that the turnover rate of APNs in the VHA system was low at 7.8% for APNs and 5.7% for CNSs, which suggests APN satisfaction in practice compared to regular staff nurses working outside the VHA system who had a turnover rate of 8.8%. Faris et al. (2010) discussed that when practice was in a shared medical appointment environment, the overall patient outcomes when managing chronic illness were better than most other models. They stated that this model; when utilised in managing hypertension, diabetes and heart failure; meant patients and families played a bigger role in their self management and decision making. The APN was a change agent with good communication skills who worked well with the team.

There are many dozens of companies that provide health insurance to Americans (De Navas-Walt et al., 2010). In recent decades there has been an effort to rein in healthcare delivery costs and two new identities emerged that have made an effort to do so: health maintenance organisations (HMO) and preferred provider organisations (PPO) are examples of groups trying to control cost; essentially by not treating patients or by limiting what will be covered. Many employers who provide their employees with health insurance will decide which HMO they offer. A HMO will have its own doctors and hospitals under contract, usually at some sort of discounted rate, and all those enrolled in these organisations will have to select from the contracted providers. Some companies pay for APN services, others may not. The traditional health insurance companies are fee-for-service, but these are becoming less common, although they do cover all services provided.

What this means for the new APN is that he or she must be aware of the business end of service provided, and this may well drive whether practice is collaborative, in a group with doctors and other specialists, or whether the APN goes into practice with only other APNs. If the APN remains within a hospital system, it may or may not separately line-item his/her services. Regular registered nurse services are not a line-item in a hospital budget or on invoices submitted to the third party payers. The APN must be knowledgeable about reimbursement issues in the particular specialty in which he/she is practicing.

The irony is that despite the plethora of groups funding health care, there are still more than 46 million people without healthcare insurance in the USA, and thus technically have no access to healthcare services unless they are willing pay out of pocket. Few can afford this. It was this glaring need that the recent healthcare reform law was trying to address.

Activity 3

Identify the advantages and disadvantages of working as an independent ANP. Besides specific malpractice insurance coverage, what other expenses are incurred in independent practice?

Prescriptive authority

Prescriptive authority includes the ordering of medication, controlled or otherwise, the ordering of laboratory and other tests, and ordering durable medical equipment. By and large prescriptive authority, which is granted by individual states, is only given to those nurses who are nurse practitioners and who have completed the courses in the 3 Ps. According Mercer Ray (2008) CRNAs do not prescribe in the administration of giving anaesthesia, although this is not necessarily true if they are managing pain. Since 2000, nurse-midwives have had some prescriptive authority in all 50 states and the District of Columbia. The 50 states differ in how they will allow NPs to prescribe medications: 'In 47 states NPs can prescribe controlled substances, although some states limit the amount the quantities prescribed or place other restrictions on this prescribing' (Mercer Ray, 2008:555). Only five states give NPs unencumbered status in relation to controlled substances: Arizona, Montana, Oregon, Washington, and Wyoming as well as the District of Columbia. All APNs who have prescriptive authority have to apply and be issued with a Federal Enforcement Agency (FEA) number, which is theirs alone and must be written on all prescriptions. In some instances the CNS has limited prescriptive authority, and the NACNS supports this as a 'discretionary option' (Mercer Ray, 2008:555), but this is usually within narrow institutional protocols.

Activity 4

If you are a nurse prescriber, what (if any) are the limitations on your prescribing privileges? Do you see a need to change these privileges? If 'yes', in what way should they be changed?

Barriers to practice

Unfortunately there remain barriers that lead to the underutilization and recognition of APNs. Many of these are politico/socio/economic. As Weilland (2008) stated, 'the factors of physician dominance, reimbursement, and state rules and regulations have created practice environments that are detrimental to full recognition of NPs as autonomous practitioners' (Weilland, 2008:345). This leads to '(a) denial of primary provider status, (b) decreased patient access to care, and (c) increased healthcare costs' (Weilland, 2008:345). What emerges from the nursing literature is that doctor dominance and resentment, and perhaps their failure to understand what APNs do, is one of the most serious threats to independent and fully autonomous APN practice. Some doctors have claimed that, compared to themselves, APNs have had too little graduate education to be able to practice independently and/or responsibly, that APNs aren't safe, do not refer appropriately and in a timely fashion, and finally, doctor supervision and collaborative practice are a must (Partin, 2009). Multiple studies in the nursing literature make clear that none of these reasons are completely valid, and in some instances the APN makes fewer errors than either the doctor or physician assistant (PA). This latter entity may be regarded as the true 'doctor extender' rather than the APN who is sometimes referred to as such. However, this has led some commentators to state that NPs have been seen as 'doctor extender' and 'cheap labour' because NPs improved physician productivity and income as each billing incident 'realized 100% reimbursement' (Weilland, 2008:347). This negates the APN as a primary care provider who emphasizes health promotion, and stresses the '"*medical*" role as a physician substitute' (Weilland, 2008:347). In many respects this is insulting, if not outright humiliating, to the autonomy of the APN. The American Academy of Family Practitioners (2006) has stated that APNs should be supervised by doctors otherwise a 'second-class system of health care' will emerge (cited by Weilland, 2008:348). Weilland also claimed that the Committee of Pediatric Workforce has also opposed independent ANP practice, prescriptive authority and reimbursement. What this suggests is that doctors retain enormous power, privilege and prestige but are fearful of any loss of economic benefits. What is ironic about this, according to Phillips (2010), who did a meta-analysis of the literature, is that NPs demonstrate high quality, safe patient care, and health outcomes and resource utilization that are equivalent to doctors. At the same time patients remain highly satisfied with NP services.

The state BON, as the licensing authority, and the rules and regulations within the State Practice Acts are highly controlling of APN practice and particularly when it comes to prescriptive authority. Thus, BONs may be seen as barriers to APN practice. This should be probably be interpreted cautiously because of the public's safety and the BON responsibility. However, Fontana's (2008) dialectical analysis of APN prescribing reveals that APNs are judiciously cautious when prescribing, and when it comes to narcotics may not or refuse to prescribe them at all. In some instances, because of fear of being prosecuted, they will ignore patients' need for narcotics to treat non-malignant chronic pain. This study suggests that innate APN caution is a barrier in itself.

Conclusion

What this chapter has demonstrated is that if you are contemplating working as an ANP as a career choice, you must be a highly informed consumer if you are to negotiate and manage your advanced practice in the USA. This can also be said of advanced practice in the UK and perhaps other countries as well. Changes in policies, rules and regulations are occurring so rapidly that remaining informed is imperative. Your career will hinge on what you select as a programme of graduate study, followed by licensure and certification requirements if you choose to practice in the USA. From there, decisions related to the type of practice you wish to pursue, whether it is within an acute care facility or in some type of non-acute care community based organisation, whether to pursue solo practice, or practice with another APN, or whether to join in a collaborative doctor practice must be examined. Reimbursement is a thorny issue, and unfortunately it has been relatively common for APNs to be practicing with a poorer population, who may or may not have healthcare insurance. Third party payers have not always reimbursed at the same rate as doctors. For NPs there is also the issue of prescriptive authority. They must be fully cognisant that this is granted by a state, and is not transferable to another state. The newly mandated federal healthcare reform has not yet made clear what the exact role is for the APN, however it does seem to offer a unique opportunity for expansion of practice. What is clear though is that APNs are satisfied with their roles in practice, and that they feel validated and valued as autonomous, independent participants in the inter-professional team. Furthermore, patients are satisfied with their services.

References

Agosta, L. J. (2009) Patient satisfaction with nurse practitioner delivered primary healthcare services. *Journal of the American Academy of Nurse Practitioner;* 21(11): 610–17.

American Academy of Family Practitioners (2006) *Guidelines on the Supervision of Certified Nurse Midwives, Nurse Practitioners and Doctors Assistants.* Available from: http://www.aafp.org. In: S. A Weilland, (2008) Reflections on independence in nurse practitioner practice. *Journal of the American Academy of Nurse Practitioners,* 221(7): 345–52. (accessed 24/03/2011).

American Academy of Nurse Practitioners (AANP) (2002) *Standards of Practice.* Available from: http://www.aanp.org (accessed 14/06/2011) In: S. A Weilland, (2008) Reflections on independence in nurse practitioner practice. *Journal of the American Academy of Nurse Practitioners.* 22(1): 345–52.

American Association of Colleges of Nursing (AACN) (2011) *The Essentials of Master's Education in Nursing.* AACN: Washington DC. Available from: http://www.aacn.nche.edu/Education/pdf/Master'sEssentials11.pdf (accessed 14/06/2011)

American Nurses Association (ANA) (2007) *Public Health Nursing. Scope and Standards of Public Health Nursing* Silver Springs, MD: American Nursing Association.

APRN Consensus Work Group and the National Council of States Boards of Nursing APRN Advisory Committee (2008) *Consensus Model for APRN Regulation: Licensure, Accreditation, Certification & Education.* Available from: https://www.ncsbn.org/7_23_08_Consensue_APRN_Final.pdf (accessed 14/06/2011).

Avery, M. D. and Howe, C. (2007) The DNP and entry into midwifery practice: An analysis. *Journal of Midwifery & Women's Health,* 52(1): 14–22.

Brooten, D., Youngblut, J. M., Deatrick, J., Naylor M. and York, R. (2003) Patient problems, advanced practice nurse (APN) interventions, time and contacts among five patient groups. *Journal of Nursing Scholarship,* 35(1): 773–79.

BHPR, (2010) *Professional Practice Indices.* Available from: http://bhpr.hrsa.gov/healthwork force/reports/scope/sope3-5htm (accessed 14/06/2011)

Cox, C. and Hall, A. (2007) Advanced Practice Role in Gastrointestinal Nursing, *Journal of Gastrointestinal Nursing,* 5(4): 26–31.

Cox, C., Gibbons, H., Whiteing, N. (2010) Advanced Practice in Ophthalmic Nursing, *Eye News Journal,* 17(1): 17–24.

De Navas-Walk, C., Proctor, B. D. and Smith, J. C. (2010) Income, Poverty and Health Insurance Coverage in the United States: 2009. Available from: http://www.census.gov/prod/2010pubs/p60–238.pdf (accessed 14/06/2011)

Deshefy-Longhi, T., Swartz, M. K. and Grey, M. (2008) Characterizing nurse practitioner practice by patient encounters: An APRNet study. *Journal of the American Academy of Nurse Practitioners,* 20(5): 281–87.

Easom, A. (2005) APN and APRN are the appropriate credentials. *Nephrology Nursing Journal.* 32(2): 86–87. Available from: http://proquest.umi.com/pqdweb?index=16&sid=1&rsch mode=1&vinst=PROD&fmt=2&s (accessed 14/06/2011)

Evans, S.T. (2010) Convenient care clinics: Making a positive change in health care. *Journal of the American Academy of Nurse Practitioners,* 22(1): 23–26.

Faris, J. A., Douglas, M. K., Maples, D. C., Berg, L. R., and Thraikill, A. (2010) Job satisfaction of advanced practice nurses in the Veterans Health Administration. *Journal of the American Academy of Nurse Practitioners,* 22(1): 35–44.

Finkelman, A. and Kenner, C. (2007) *Teaching IOM: Implications of the Institute of Medicine Reports for Nursing Education.* 2nd Ed. Silver Springs MD: American Nurses Association.

Fontana, J. S. (2008) The social and political forces affecting prescribing practices for chronic pain. *Journal of Professional Nursing,* 24(1): 30–35.

Goudreau, K. A., Clark, A., Fulton, J. and Sendelbach, S. (2007) A vision of the future for clinical nurse specialists. *Clinical Nurse Specialist,* 21(6): 310–20.

Hauer, K. E., Durning, S. J., Kernan, W. N., Fagin, M. J. and O'Sullivan, P. S. (2008) Factors associated with medical students' career choices regarding internal medicine. *Journal of the American Medical Association,* 300(10): 1154–64.

He, W., Sengupta, M., Velkoff, V. and DeBarros, K. (2005) *Current Population Reports: 65 + in the United States.* Washington, DC: US Census Bureau, Government Printing Office. In: J. M. Stanley, K. E. Werner and K. Apple. (Eds), 2009. Positioning advanced practice registered nurses for health care reform: consensus on APRN regulation. *Journal of Professional Nursing,* 25(6): 340–48.

Institute of Medicine (1999) *To Err is Human.* Washington, DC: The National Academies Press.

—— (2001) *Crossing the Quality Chasm.* Washington, DC: The National Academies Press.

—— (2003a) *Priority Areas for National Action: Transforming Healthcare Quality.* Washington, DC: The National Academies Press.

—— (2003b) *Future of the Public's Health in the 21st Century.* Washington, DC: The National Academies Press.

—— (2003c) *Who will Keep the Public Healthy?* Washington, DC: The National Academies Press.

Kleinpell, R. M., Hravnak, M., Hinch, B., and Llewellyn, J. (2008) Developing advanced practice nursing credentialing model for acute care facilities. *Nursing Administration Quarterly,* 32(4): 279–87.

Mercer Ray, M. (2008) Advanced practice registered nurse policy issues in today's health care climate. *Journal of Emergency Nursing,* 34(6): 555–57.

National Organisation of Nurse Practitioner Faculties Domains and Core Competencies of Nurse Practitioner Practice (2006) Available from: http://nonpf.com/associations/10789/files/DomainsandCoreComps2006.pdf (accessed 14/06/2011).

Nursing and Midwifery Council (2005) *Annex 1 Domains of Practice and Competencies, NMC Consultation on a Proposed Framework for Post-registration Nursing.* London: NMC.

Partin, B. (2009) APRN/Physician collaboration: A call to action. *Nurse Practitioner*, 34(1): 6. Available from: http://proquest.umi.com/pqdweb?index=1&sid=1&srchmode=1&vinst=PROD&fmt=2&st (accessed 16/03/2010).

Patient Health Protection and Affordable Care Law and Health Care and Education Reconciliation Practice Act. (March 2010) *Patient Health Protection and Affordable Care Law* and *Health Care and Education Reconciliation Practice Act*, Available from: http://www.gpo.gov/fdsys/pkg/BILLS-111hr3590enr/pdf/BILLS-111hr3590enr.pdf (accessed 14/06/2011).

Phillips. (2010). 22nd Annual Legislative Update: Regulatory and legislative successes of ARPNs *The Nurse Practitioner*, 35(1): 24–47. www.tnpj.com.

Public Health Law 111–148, (2011). Available from: http://www.gpo.gov/fdsys/pkg/PLAW-111publ148/pdf/PLAW-111publ148.pdf (accessed 14/06/2011)

Royal College of Nursing (2010a) *Advanced Nurse Practitioners – An RCN Guide to the Advanced Nurse Practitioner Role, Competences and Programme* Accreditation. Available from: http://www.rcn.org.uk/__data/assets/pdf_file/0003/146478/003207.pdf (accessed 14/06/2011).

Stanley, J. M., Werner, K. E. and Apple, K. (2009) Positioning advanced practice registered nurses for health care reform: Consensus on APRN regulation. *Journal of Professional Nursing*, 25(6): 340–48.

Stewart, J. G., McNulty, R. M., Quinn Griffin, A. T. and Fitzpatrick, J. J. (2010) Psychological empowerment and structural empowerment among nurse practitioners. *Journal of the American Academy of Nurse Practitioners*, 22(1): 27–34.

Tuite, P. K. and George, E. L. (2010) The role of the clinical nurse specialist in facilitating evidence-based practice within a university setting. *Critical Care Nursing Quarterly*, 33(2): 117–25.

Upvall. M. J. and Ptachcinski, R. J. (2007) The journey to the DNP programme and beyond: What we can learn from pharmacy? *Journal of Professional Nursing*, 23(5): 316–21.

Watts, S., Gee, J., O'Day, M. E., Schaub, K., Lawrence, R., Aron, D. and Kirsh, S. (2009) *Journal of the American Academy of Nurse Practitioners*, 21(3): 167–72.

Weilland, S. A. (2008) Reflections on independence in nurse practitioner practice. *Journal of the American Academy of Nurse Practitioners*, 22(1): 345–52.

Section III **Leadership: The Professional Role**

Chapter 7 **Professionalism in Advanced Practice: The professional role**

Carol L. Cox

Introduction

Professionalism is defined as 'the conduct, aims, or qualities that characterise or mark a profession or a professional person' (Merriam-Webster, 2003:991). 'In assuming a professional role, one conforms to the technical or ethical standards of a profession exhibiting a courteous, conscientious and generally businesslike manner in the workplace' (Merriam-Webster, 2003:991).

According to Brehm et al. (2006), the concept of professionalism is multifaceted. Professionalism may be divided into three components or categories which are: professional parameters, professional behaviours and professional responsibilities (Bossers et al., 1999). Professional parameters include legal and ethical issues whilst professional behaviours are related to discipline-related knowledge and skills, relationships with clients and colleagues in which collaboration and collegiality become essential components and an acceptable appearance and attitude. Finally professional responsibilities relate to a responsibility to one's profession, to oneself, clients, employers and the community. Individuals must develop the full spectrum of characteristics, attitudes and behaviours including a life-long commitment to professionalism if one is to be regarded as a professional (Brehm et al., 2006; Hammer et al., 2003).

Learning outcomes

At the conclusion of this chapter you will be able to:

- Describe the elements of professionalism associated with clinical/direct care advanced practice
- Discuss professionalism in relation to leadership and collaborative advanced practice

- Relate professionalism to improving quality and developing advanced practice
- Formulate plans for developing self and others at an advanced practice level.

Background

The Council for Healthcare Regulatory Excellence (CHRE, 2009) confirmed the need for a nationally agreed set of standards for advanced level practice in nursing. Since that event it has been recognised that all professions involved in direct care delivery working at an advanced level of practice, regardless of the area of practice, setting or client group should be practicing to the same level of standards. In November 2010, the Department of Health (DoH) for England under the auspices of the Chief Nursing Officer for England, Dame Christine Beasley, published its definitive position statement on Advanced Level Nursing. In the document it is indicated that the purpose of the statement is to 'improve understanding of advanced level practice, and will act as an aid to assist practitioners, commissioners, educators, service and workforce planners achieve their aim of building services focused on improving outcomes and experiences for patients' (DoH, 2010:2). The position statement is intended to be used as a benchmark that will enhance patient safety and the delivery of high quality care. Without question, this document is an indication of standards associated with professionalism. In this chapter the essential elements associated with professionalism at an advanced practice level will be addressed. These elements are explicated in the DoH (2010) position statement and for the purpose of this chapter will be associated with all healthcare professions involved in the delivery of care to patients. The nationally agreed elements of advanced practice are described under four themes. These themes are:

> Clinical/direct care practice;
> Leadership and collaborative practice;
> Improving quality and developing practice; and
> Developing self and others.

> (DoH, 2010:5)

Linked to each theme are elements associated with advanced practice. These elements should be regarded as a minimum threshold that demonstrates the essential attributes of professionalism. In relation to professionalism, it can be seen that professionalism involves respect for patients and coworkers, knowledge of discipline, accountability, flexibility, trustworthiness, ethical behaviour, teamwork, confidentiality, honesty and reliability (Brehm at al, 2006). Furthermore, in accordance with the position statement on advanced practice, it can be seen that professionalism is underpinned by the assumptions that all healthcare professionals:

- take personal responsibility for their actions and omissions and fully recognise their personal accountability;
- are able to make sound decisions about their ongoing personal and professional development; practising within the scope of their personal professional competence and extending this scope as appropriate; delegating aspects of care to others and accepting responsibility and accountability for such delegation; and working harmoniously and effectively with colleagues, patients and clients and their carers, families and friends; and
- are expected to conduct themselves and practice within an ethical framework based upon respect for the well-being and safety of patients and clients.

(DoH, 2010:5)

Elements of professionalism associated with clinical/direct care advanced practice

Professionalism in advanced clinical practice

Professionalism can be readily recognised in the definition of advanced level nursing published by the Department of Health (2010). According to the Department of Health (2010:7), at an advanced practice level, the healthcare professional is 'deeply involved in promoting public health and well-being.' These professionals 'understand the implications of the social, economic and political context of healthcare and their professional and clinical judgement are demonstrated in the expert nature of their practice and depth of their knowledge' (DoH 2010:7). Furthermore, 'patients, clients and other professionals acknowledge their highly developed and extensive knowledge in areas such as diagnostics, therapeutics, the biological, social and epidemiological sciences and pharmacology and their enhanced skills in consultation and clinical decision-making' (DoH 2010:7). Healthcare professionals working at an advanced practice level use 'complex reasoning, critical thinking, reflection and analysis to inform their assessment, clinical judgements and decisions. They are able to apply knowledge and skills to a broad range of clinically and professionally challenging and complex situations' (DoH 2010:7).

The Nursing and Midwifery Council (NMC, 2010:1) produced a consultation document on advanced practice for nurses in 2005 in which it indicated that these nurses:

- Take a comprehensive patient history
- Carry out physical examinations
- Use their expert knowledge and clinical judgement to identify the potential diagnosis
- Refer patients for investigations where appropriate
- Make a final diagnosis
- Decide on and carry out treatment, including the prescribing of medicines, or refer patients to an appropriate specialist
- Use their extensive practice experience to plan and provide skilled and competent care to meet patients' health and social care needs, involving other members of the health care team as appropriate;
- Ensure the provision of continuity of care including follow-up visits
- Assess and evaluate, with patients, the effectiveness of the treatment and care provided and make changes as needed
- Work independently, although often as part of a health care team
- Provide leadership
- Make sure that each patient's treatment and care is based on best practice.

(NMC, 2010)

As of February 2006, it was agreed that these were the definitive activities of the advanced nurse practitioner. In addition it indicated that 'Advanced nurse practitioners are highly experienced and educated members of the care team who are able to diagnose and treat your health care needs or refer you to an appropriate specialist if needed' (NMC, 2010:1). Aspects of these activities and its definition of the advanced nurse practitioner can be seen as defining characteristics of all advanced practitioners in relation to attributes of professionalism in practice. Table 7.1 shows the NMC (2010) competencies associated with the practice element of the professional role that were originally published in 2005.

It is apparent from the competencies listed in Table 7.1 that there is a blending of practice, education and research into the clinical role. The advanced healthcare practitioner is functioning as a co-ordinator, consultant, coach, advocate, administrator, educator, researcher, role model and leader in addition to providing direct patient care. How then does one develop this level of expertise?

TABLE 7.1   Nursing and Midwifery Council Competencies in the Professional Role Related to Practice

---

Competencies

Develops and implements the advanced nurse practitioner role

1   Uses evidence and research to implement the role.
2   Functions in a variety of role dimensions: healthcare provider, coordinator, consultant, educator, coach, advocate, administrator, researcher, role model and leader.
3   Interprets and markets the role to the public, legislators, policy-maker, and other healthcare professions.

Directs care

1   Prioritises, coordinates, and meets multiple needs for culturally diverse patients.
2   Uses sound judgement in assessing conflicting priorities and needs.
3   Builds and maintains a therapeutic team to provide optimum therapy.
4   Obtains specialist and referral care for patients while remaining the primary care provider.
5   Acts as an advocate for the patient to ensure health needs are met consistent with patients' wishes.
6   Consults with other healthcare providers and public/independent agencies.
7   Incorporates current technology appropriately in care delivery.
8   Uses information systems to support decision-making and to improve care.

(NMC, 2010:17 'Consultation Document')

Learning the professional role

Professionalism is informally learned through role modelling by other professionals, instructors and preceptors. What is critical within the process of learning a professional role is assimilation of the values and behaviours associated with the discipline being acquired. Health professionals should be taught to coordinate, collaborate and communicate with one another in interdisciplinary teams so that appropriate clinical decisions are made and ethical dilemmas are solved (Brehm et al., 2006; Institute of Medicine, Committee on Quality of Health Care in America, 2001; Cloonan et al., 1999). To achieve this, it involves the integration of discipline-specific knowledge, skills and perspectives. In so doing, optimal patient care that encompasses the expertise of each health professional can be delivered (Brehm et al., 2006; Brennan, 2002). Interdisciplinary learning opportunities enhance understanding and appreciation of one's profession and its potential contributions to the health care team.

Activity 1

Identify aspects of your practice in which you have learned to practice at an advanced practice level through the role modelling of others.

Answer the following questions:

- How do you function as a role model for others?
- Do you role model in same way as your instructors and preceptors have role modelled for you?
- What aspects of role modelling come easily to you?
- What aspects of role modelling are difficult for you and how can you overcome these difficulties?

Tip for helping others learn

The goals of learning are to stress the importance of professionalism in the clinical environment, to provide information in relation to the various health disciplines and interdisciplinary teams that are involved in healthcare. One good way to learn about what is appropriate is to consider what is *not* appropriate. This can be initiated through role play in which clinically-based scenarios are enacted in which non-professional behaviours, skills and attitudes are reviewed. Field experience provides opportunities to gain insight into the roles and responsibilities of other health professionals. Here, professional traits and behaviours can be observed in a natural setting. The learner can consider how their own discipline might contribute to care in the context in which healthcare is being delivered.

Professionalism in relation to leadership and collaborative advanced practice

Leadership and collaboration

Collaborating with others sounds easy on the face of it. However, with diverse interests in practice disciplines and competing demands for the patient's or client's healthcare regimen it is possible to come into conflict regarding the best plan of care for the patient/client. Plochg et al. (2009:2) state that 'As the status of medical work is, at least in part, competitive, professionalization is linked to the pursuit of internal control over medical work and outperforming rival specialities.' Brennan (2002) and Plochg et al., (2009) indicate that a commitment must be made to working with others to ensure that health care teams working within the healthcare environment produce the best possible outcomes for patients. This means taking up the banner to lead systematic analyses of quality care and working with others to develop better methods of care (Katz el al, 2007). According to the Department of Health (2010), this involves providing consultancy services to one's own and other professions in relation to therapeutic interventions and practice and service development. It also means working 'across professional, organisational and system boundaries and proactively developing and sustaining new partnerships and networks to influence and improve health, outcomes and healthcare delivery systems' (DoH 2010:10).

Within the context of leadership, the Department of Health (2010) has also been clear that the advanced practice practitioner engages stakeholders and uses high-level negotiating and influencing skills in order to develop and improve practice. Part of this can come about through recognition of a need for change. However, moving forward to generate practice innovations and then leading on practice and service redesign solutions that meet the needs of patients/clients and the service in better ways sometimes means changing the perspective on relationships between doctors, managers and other healthcare clinicians. The perspective is changed to ensure that the improvements recommended are based on careful research and data that has been mediated by continuous quality improvement methods (Brennan, 2002). Generating practice innovations and leading on practice and service redesign are essential components of the advanced practice practitioner's remit.

Over the past decade, healthcare reform has brought about a change in the structure of healthcare, both in the primary care and secondary care sector. Considerable progress has been made in making healthcare more accessible to patients and moving healthcare management to the control of non-doctor health system managers (Taylor, 1996). This places the advanced practice practitioner in an ideal position to manage a multidisciplinary healthcare team. Leading a multidisciplinary healthcare team requires considerable tact, discretionary and experiential expertise and an inherent component of clinical practice (Plochg et al., 2009). Expertise and knowledge are required to navigate patients through systems, ensure that patients experience not only better health outcomes but also that costs associated with delivering healthcare are controlled effectively. Knowledge of health policy and how systems relate between the primary and secondary care sector is invaluable. Additionally active involvement in one's professional organisation/college can provide much-needed guidance and support to professionals undertaking leadership positions. Table 7.2 shows the NMC (2010) competencies associated with the leadership element of the professional role that were originally published in 2005.

TABLE 7.2 Nursing and Midwifery Council Competencies in the Professional Role Related to Leadership

Competencies

Provides leadership

1   Is actively involved in a professional association.
2   Evaluates implications of contemporary health policy on health care providers and consumers.
3   Participates in legislative and policy-making activities that influence an advanced level of nursing practice and the health of communities.
4   Advocates for access to quality, cost-effective health care.
5   Evaluates the relationship between community/public health issues and social problems as they impact on the health care of patients (poverty, literacy, violence, etc.).
6   Actively engages in continuous professional development and maintains a suitable record of this development.

(NMC, 2010:17 'Consultation Document')

Activity 2

Consider your involvement in the healthcare team. Are you influencing change? Are you leading a team? If 'no' is your response, what do you need to do to increase the leadership components of your professional role?

Construct a plan of action for a healthcare innovation that you think requires introduction in your healthcare setting. How feasible is it to implement this plan of action? What negotiating skills do you need to bring about introduction of the innovation?

Improving quality, developing practice, self and others

Autonomous practice, self-direction and self regulation

Essential components of professionalism within the context of advanced practice include autonomous practice, self-direction, self-regulation and proactive involvement in the development of strategies and the undertaking of activities that monitor and improve the quality of healthcare and the effectiveness of one's own and others' practice (DoH, 2010). The aim of professional self-regulation is to make individual practitioners more accountable to their peers (van Herk et al., 2001; Klein, 1998; 1997). Clinical autonomy can be considered the core of professional autonomy (van Herk et al., 2001).

Clinical or technical autonomy is defined as the right of the profession to set its own standards and control clinical performance (Elston, 1991). As an autonomous advanced practice practitioner, the healthcare professional continually assesses and monitors risk in relation to their own and others' practice and challenges others about wider risk factors (DoH, 2010). These individuals 'plan and seize opportunities to generate and apply new knowledge to their own and others' practice in structured ways which are capable of evaluation' (DoH, 2010:11) through clinical audit and other mechanisms.

Brennan (2002), Katz et al. (2007) and Plochg et al. (2009) indicate that there is a new civic professionalism that is calling for systematic quality measurement and improvement. Brennan (2002:976) further indicates that an 'observer of the past 20 years of our health system might remark that professionalism has been eclipsed somewhat as a source of reform for health care institutions . . . by the market . . . and regulatory approaches sponsored by the government. The mandates of professional obligations are rarely used (anymore) to justify reform.' However this has not been the case traditionally, nor should it be the only route recognised as providing the platform for quality care. The healthcare professions are defined as occupations controlling specific knowledge within their disciplines and hence possessing specific activities in commerce (Brennan, 2002) that have been and are held to higher expectations by the public. As such there is a professional obligation to take seriously the mandate of promoting quality care. The Department of Health (2010) indicates that advanced practice practitioners 'continually evaluate and audit the practice of self and others at individual and systems levels, selecting and applying valid and reliable approaches and methods which are appropriate to needs and context, and acting on the findings' (DoH, 2010:10). They further 'strive constantly to improve practice and health outcomes so that they are consistent with or better than national and international standards through

145

initiating, facilitating and leading change at individual, team, organisational and system levels' (DoH 2010:10).

It may be argued that professionalism can be considered a platform for reform of the healthcare system and a means of delivering high quality care. It may also be argued that professionalism should be understood as an ideology of social reform (Brennan, 2002; McGlynn and Brook, 2001). As an alternative to market demand and government regulatory approaches, professionalism can infuse social responsibility (Sullivan, 1999) into the healthcare system. In this perspective advanced practice practitioners must been seen as advocates for their patients/clients and carers as well. As responsible autonomous practitioners they must advocate for and on behalf of the community of patients and their interests.

Civic professionalism

The principles underlying civic professionalism have derived from traditional professional values and extend the accountability of advanced practice to a social contract with the public. In this model, under the direction of the advanced practice practitioner, patients take an active role in shaping health care delivery (Katz et al., 2007). Brennan (2002:979) indicates that 'Civic professionalism's movement from individual obligation to social obligation can help provide the intellectual base for treating health as a system.' Civic professionalism in relation to quality improvements mandates a team effort in today's health care organisations.

The Department of Health (2010:9) is clear that as autonomous and self-directed professionals, advanced practice practitioners 'identify and implement systems to promote their contribution and demonstrate the impact of advanced level practice to the healthcare team and the wider health and social care sector'. Therefore there must be a commitment to professional competence, a commitment to lifelong learning through continuous professional development and recertification, a commitment to establishing trust with patients and fostering honesty with patients; particularly when errors occur in health care (Katz et al., 2007). In relation to civic professional norms, there is a requirement that patients be informed promptly so that a trusting relationship is maintained between the advanced practice practitioner and the patient/client and their carers.

In addition, it is essential that a commitment for improving the quality of care is undertaken. Professionalism mandates that the advanced practice practitioner maintains their clinical competence and also works with other professionals to ensure that the best possible outcomes are produced for patients within the context of all health care settings – be it primary, secondary or tertiary care. In the United Kingdom and in the United States of America as well as many other countries there is a Patient Charter indicating that quality care will be provided and maintained.

Finally, in consideration of professionalism, as advanced practice practitioners there is an obligation to act as role models, to actively participate in interdisciplinary teams, to actively use data and to promote the use of evidence-based practice. Poor-quality care must be reported when it occurs and appropriate use of quality systems must be utilised in an attempt to prevent inappropriate care (Katz et al., 2007).

Professionalism represents a contract between highly trained professionals and the public (Brennan, 2002). This contract creates special responsibilities; the most critical being promoting quality of care. Modern quality improvement requires a team effort. This means working together to place patient welfare at his or her highest value (Brennan, 2002) and to enhance the patient experience. Quality of care is impacted and professionalism is lost in instances of complacency, arrogance, inability to self-regulate, a 'head in the sand' syndrome and poor leadership (Hughes, 2006). Factors associated with a decline in professionalism include a perspective of the locus of control over practice being external to the individual and a loss of discretion (Harrison and Ahmad, 2000).

Activity 3

Consider how you can be involved in developing systems of better quality when your time is limited, due to the expansive number of patients you are responsible for managing.

Tip regarding civic professionalism

Society at large defines quality in terms of the health care organisation promoting health and preventing error. Your professional role as an advanced practice practitioner is to maintain integrity, compassion, excellence, continuous quality improvement and working in partnership with the health care team.

Assessment of professionalism

Measuring professionalism is a difficult process. According to Hodges et al. (2009) there is no specific method that has emerged as the definitive means of assessing professionalism. Literature reviews demonstrate a lack of current evidence when measuring attitudes related to professionalism in medical and other healthcare professions educational processes. In medical education within the past 25 years (as of 2004), 88 different methods of assessing professionalism have been proposed (Lynch et al., 2004). Outside of medical education the landscape for assessing professionalism becomes more bereft. Generally competency assessment frameworks are espoused as a mechanism for assessing aspects of professionalism (Plochg et al., 2009; Ruth et al., 2008; Katz et al., 2007), however these frameworks lack specifics and are external mechanisms with limited impact on changing behaviour.

A sign of professionalism is recognition of lapses in professional judgement. However determining the best method of assessing recognition and subsequent professionalism can be tortuous. Identification of the responsibilities of the healthcare professional is a necessary step in the process of assessment and remediation (Welbourn and Theodore, 2010). Reflection has been shown to be highly important in the development of professional behaviours (Johns, 2010; Hodges et al., 2009). Lapses in professional judgement can be explored through reflection in practice; thus leading to significant development of professional behaviour.

When advanced practice practitioners recognise through reflection that there has been a lapse in professional judgement and demonstrate guilt and remorse for their actions there is potential for remedial action. They can acknowledge a lack of knowledge and or skill. This action is termed 'acceptance' (Hodges et al., 2009). Denial of a fault in themselves is associated with feelings of the situation being out of their control. This action is termed 'rejection' (Hodges et al., 2009) and can have serious consequences in terms of patient-health outcomes. Reporting and reflecting is a sign of maturity in the professional. Reporting and reflecting demonstrate acceptance. Reflection provides a strong platform from which lapses in professional behaviour can be improved and promote positive changes. The absence of reflection and/or the inability to respond adequately to events is an indicator of unprofessional behaviour (Hodges et al., 2009). 'Report and Reflect' (Hodges et al., 2009:4) is a system of incident reporting and is a recognised mechanism for individuals to use within the context of their professional practice.

Activity 4

Critical incident reports are enhanced when combined with reflection (Hodges et al., 2009). How would you report and reflect on a critical incident that has occurred in your practice? Can you indicate an incident of 'acceptance'? Can you indicate an incident that was an occasion of 'rejection'? If the incident was one of 'rejection', how would you, following reflection address this incident now?

Tip about patient welfare

As professionals, advanced practice practitioners place patient welfare as their highest value.

Commitment to lifelong learning (Brennan, 2002)

'Academic courses and seminars that require socialization and collaboration across disciplines should address professionalism, confidence in discipline specific knowledge and skills, and respect for the actual and potential contributions of the participating disciplines to optimal health care. Small group activities are effective teaching strategies that emphasise the importance of collaboration, collegiality, professionalism, decision making, and problem solving among team members' (Brehm et al., 2006:5). To promote learning about how to collaborate across disciplines those who act as role models, instructors and preceptors must be cognisant of their own professional values and beliefs as well as those from other disciplines. They must be open and honest in their communication of their professional knowledge, skills and attitudes to those learning from them (Brehm et al., 2006; Brennan, 2002; Glen, 1999).

Activity 5

Consider how your professional developments are being addressed. Are you undertaking academic courses that develop or enhance your advanced practice knowledge and skills?

Indicate how you will engage others in clinical seminars designed to promote patients health and well-being.

> ## Tip Regarding the Maintenance of Your Professional Registration
>
> Most regulatory bodies (e.g., the Nursing and Midwifery Council, the Healthcare Professions Council and the State Boards of Nursing) require thorough on-going continuous professional development through certificate and recertification programmes. Re-examination of practice is essential for validation of competent professional practice.

According to the Department of Health (2010:6), the learning and development requirements of healthcare professionals at an advanced practice level should be 'identified and supported through individual performance review, appraisal and revalidation requirements on an ongoing basis and alongside a robust clinical supervision framework.' Part of professionalism is the responsibility to continuously assess and develop one's practice.

Protecting the public

'Maintaining and improving standards of service and care are central to professionalism in health care. The origins of the bodies that now represent and regulate medicine, nursing, pharmacy, and other professions in the health care sector are closely related to the need to protect the public from "quackery" and the excesses of competition. This is appropriate in a service where users – patients are often profoundly vulnerable' (Taylor, 1996:312). Although this statement was written in 1996, it has resonance for advanced practice practitioners today. There have been a plethora of papers and standards of practice (Refer to the Health Professions Council and the Nursing and Midwifery Council Standards of Practice as examples) written to protect the public from potential harm that can occur in the health care system. There have also been a plethora of quality measures instituted in the health care system. These strong institutional structures underpin health care professionalism (Taylor, 1996). However they do not substitute for the ethical values and beliefs that every advanced practice practitioner should embrace as a fundamental of their professionalism. As advocates for patients, the advanced practice practitioner has a responsibility to work toward eliminating neglect and inadequate care. Much of this can be accomplished as indicated previously in this chapter. Primarily this is accomplished by working effectively with one's clinical colleagues in the interests of patients (Ruth et al., 2008).

By emphasising prevention and health promotion the well-being of patients can be enhanced. By working effectively – proactively within the healthcare team – potential is increased to ameliorate social health problems. As a professional engaging in advanced practice, there is a moral obligation to respect patients as persons, to encourage patients' involvement in the delivery of care and to ensure that their privacy and dignity are maintained.

Conclusion

The increasing complexity of care, coordination of multiple patient needs, and delivery of care across clinical environments means that professionalism is an essential ingredient for positive clinical outcomes. Part of professionalism involves teamwork. Teamwork amongst disciplines should be stressed in order to ease the transition from a basic professional role to an advanced practice professional role. This endeavour will enhance the advanced practice practitioner's effectiveness as a member of the health care team. This chapter has indicated that as professionals, one must report poor quality of care when it occurs. One must advocate for the use of appropriate systems in all areas where healthcare is provided. Finally, as an advanced practice practitioner one must actively promote patient and carer involvement in the development, delivery and evaluation of care.

References

Bossers, A., Kernaghan, J., Hodgins, L., Merla, L., O'Connor, C. and Van Kessel, M. (1999) Defining and developing professionalism. *Canadian Journal of Occupational Therapy*, 66(3): 16–21.

Brehm, B., Breen, P., Brown, B., Long, L., Smith, R., Wall, A. and Warren, N. (2006) Instructional design and assessment: An interdisciplinary approach to introducing professionalism, *American Journal of Pharmaceutical Education* 70(4): 1–5.

Brennan, R. (2002) Physicians' Professional Responsibility to Improve the Quality of Care. *Academic Medicine*, 77(10): 973–80.

CHRE (2009) *Advanced Practice: Report to the four UK Health Departments*. Unique ID 17-2008. Council for Healthcare Regulatory Excellence. Available from: www.chre.org.uk/_img/pics/library/090709_Advanced_Practice_report_FINAL.pdf (accessed 14/06/2011)

Cloonan, P., David, F. and Burnett, C. (1999) Interdisciplinary education in clinical ethics: a work in progress. *Holistic Nurse Practitioner* 13(2): 12–19.

DoH (2010) *Advanced Level Nursing: A Position Statement*. Department of Health, 403775, 10 November 2010. London: Produced by COI for the Department of Health. Available from: www.dh.gov.uk/publications (accessed 10/01/11).

Elston, M. (1991) The politics of professional power, medicine in a changing health service, in Gabe, J., Calnan, M. and Bury, M. (Eds), *The Sociology of the Heatlh Service*. London: Routledge.

Glen, S. (1999) Educating for interprofessional collaboration: teaching about values. *Nursing Ethics*, 6(3): 202–13.

Hammer, D., Berger, B. and Beadsley, R. (2003) Student professionalism. *American Journal of Pharm Education* 67(3): 1–29.

Harrison, S. and Ahmad, W. (2000) Medical autonomy and the UK state 1975 to 2025. *Sociology* 34(1): 129–46.

Hodges, D., McLachlan, J. and Finn, G. (2009) Exploring reflective 'critical incident' documentation of professionalism lapses in medical undergraduate setting. *BMC Medical Education*, 9(44): 1–5.

Hughes, G. (2006) Medical professionalism in the 21st century; how do we stack up? *Journal of Emergency Medicine*, 23(4):44.

Institute of Medicine, Committee on Quality of Health Care in America (2001) *Crossing the Quality Chasm: A New Health System for the 21st Century.* Washington, D.C.: National Academy Press.

Johns, C. (2010) *Clinical Supervision: Reflective practice; learning through experience*, in Cox, C. and Hill, M. (Eds), *Professional Issues in Primary Care*, Chapter 11. Oxford: Wiley-Blackwell pp: 173–85.

Katz, J., Kessler, C., O'Connell, A. and Levine, S. (2007) Professionalism and Evolving Concepts of Quality. *Society of General Internal Medicine*, 22(1): 137–39.

Klein, R. (1998) *Regulating the Medical Profession: Doctors and the Public Interest 1997/1998.* Health Care UK, London: Kings Fund pp: 152–63.

—— (1997) *The New Politics of the NHS.* London: Longman.

Lynch, D., Surdyk, P. and Eiser A. (2004) Assessing professionalism: a review of the literature. *Medical Teacher*, 26(4): 366–73.

McGlynn, E. and Brook, R. (2001) Keeping quality on the policy agenda. *Health Aff.* 20(3): 82–90.

Merriam-Webster's Collegiate Dictionary (2003) *Merriam-Webster's Collegiate Dictionary*, 11th Edition, Springfield Massachusetts: Merriam-Webster, Incorporated.

NMC (2010) Consultation Document http://www.nmc-uk.org/Get-involved/Consultations/Past-consultations/By-year/The-proposed-framework-for-the-standard-for-post-registration-nursing---February-2005/ (accessed 14/06/2011)

Plochg, T., Klazinga, N. and Starfield, B. (2009) Transforming medical professionalism to fit changing health needs. *BMC Medicine*, 7(64): 1–7.

Ruth, B., Sisco, S., Wyatt, J., Bachman, S. and Piper, T. (2008) Public Health and Social Work: Training Dual Professionals for the Contemporary Workplace. *Public Health Reports*, 2(123): 71–77.

Sullivan, W. (1999) What is left of professionalism after managed care? *Hastings Centre Rep.* 29(2): 7–13.

Taylor, D. (1996) Quality and professionalism in health care: a review of current initiatives in the NHS. *BMJ* 312(7031): 626–29.

Van Herk, R., Klazinga, N. and Schepers, R. (2001) Medical audit: threat or opportunity for the medical profession. A comprehensive study of medical audit among medical specialists in general hospitals in the Netherlands and England, 1970 – 1999. *The Lancet*, 305(7905): 511–13.

Welbourn, D. and Theodore, C. (2010) *Revalidation – demonstrating continuing fitness to practice.* Final Report to the Nursing and Midwifery Council, 29 June 2010. London: Matrix Knowledge Ltd.

Chapter 8 Clinical Effectiveness

Nicola Whiteing

Introduction

The need for advanced practitioners has become acute and with diminishing numbers of medical and Allied Health Professionals (AHPs) there are implications for the extension of practice and the assumption of advanced practice roles such as Advanced Nurse Practitioners (ANP), Nurse Consultants (Cox, 2010a) and extended scope physiotherapists. The enthusiasm and speed of workforce planning teams to implement advanced practitioner roles has brought with it variances in role definitions and preparation of staff to undertake such roles. It is therefore imperative both to patients and the organisation that outcomes of care are obtained and evaluated in measuring and ensuring clinical effectiveness.

Whilst clinical effectiveness is an area that has important implications for patient care it is also important for individual staff development (Cox and Ahluwalia, 2000). As such, this chapter will explore ways in which outcomes related to clinical effectiveness can be obtained, implemented and evaluated for both the effectiveness of care delivery and also the role of the advanced practitioner. Key areas including evidence-based practice, audit, research, patient satisfaction, the case manager role and continuing professional development will be explored.

Learning outcomes

At the conclusion of this chapter you will be able to:

* Understand the importance of clinical effectiveness and to be able to articulate its three elements
* Discuss ways in which the advanced practitioner can become involved in the implementation of evidence-based practice
* Discuss the role of the advanced practitioner as a case manager drawing on relevant domains and competencies of practice

- Demonstrate an awareness of a variety of tools to enable collection of evaluative data on which to review practice, discussing their advantages and disadvantages
- Articulate ways in which the advanced practitioner can address continuing professional development activities for the benefit of the organisation and the individual.

Background

Evidence on which to base best practice is generated through measurement of clinical effectiveness, and is part of the evaluation process that demonstrates whether changes to practice are appropriate, effective and efficient (Rycroft-Malone et al., 2002). Various definitions of clinical effectiveness exist but perhaps the most commonly cited is that of the NHS Executive:

> Clinical effectiveness is demonstrated when specific clinical interventions do what they are intended to do, which is to maintain and improve health while securing the greatest possible health gain from available resources.
>
> NHS Executive (1996:45).

Clinical effectiveness has three distinctive parts (Cranston, 2002):

- Obtaining the evidence
- Implementing the evidence
- Evaluating the impact of the changed practice.

The National Health Service (NHS) Plan (DoH, 2000a) states that the NHS must be driven by a cycle of continuous quality improvement and alongside the introduction of clinical governance the government's determination is reflected to ensure high quality healthcare. Clinical governance encompasses everything that helps to maintain and improve high standards of patient care, providing the advanced practitioner with a framework to ensure that quality of care is demonstrable and applicable to all providers and disciplines through its various components including: clinical effectiveness, risk management, information technology, practice development (lifelong learning), clinical audit, health and safety and research and development. Evidence-based practice (EBP) is concerned with changing clinical practice to improve patient care (Levin and Feldman, 2006) and is a key component of clinical governance. Advanced practitioners should ensure their contribution to clinical governance reports and the compilation of the services clinical governance portfolio by outlining existing achievements in addition to short-, medium- and long-term planned goals for the advanced practice service.

There is mounting pressure being exerted to ensure that healthcare delivery is evidence-based and clinically effective. EBP enhances the healthcare environment and facilitates competent clinical practice, innovation and a commitment to progressing a profession (DeBourgh, 2001). Through the integration of clinical expertise and the best available external evidence from good research studies, the advanced practitioner is given confidence that their clinical, managerial and educational interventions are informed by a current and appropriate knowledge base (Cranston, 2002). Using research in practice is not a new notion (Whiteing, 2008) however there is now more of an emphasis on a systematic approach to its analysis, use of information to influence practice and the analysis and evaluation of outcomes on patient care (Munro, 2004). The concept of EBP has been driven though a number of government documents which aim for a health service in which clinical, managerial and policy decisions are no longer based on tradition or ritual but on sound and pertinent information. The evolution of National Service Frameworks (NSFs) and the National Institute of Clinical Excellence (NICE) all contribute to providing evidence on best practice. With EBP being high on the healthcare agenda the advanced practitioner must develop necessary skills in this area (Griffiths, 2003). This includes steps on how to search for evidence effectively (Burke et al., 2005) and learn how to integrate EBP into their caring practice (Fineout-Overholt et al., 2005). This will enable practice to become more appropriate, timely and acceptable to the patient, the wider inter-disciplinary team and the organisation. The advanced practitioner is in an ideal position to lead on the development and implementation of EBP through actively participating in the design, implementation and evaluation of changes made to healthcare systems. It is necessary for the advanced practitioner to promote EBP within the organisation as a way of improving the quality of patient care (DeBourgh, 2001). Table 8.1 illustrates a number of ways in which the advanced practitioner can begin to get involved in the implementation of EBP and assist others in doing so.

Often the current practice is not what is known to be best practice; indeed, there is a real challenge in implementing a change in practice. Practitioners have a duty to deliver evidence based practice but they often do not understand the factors that influence implementation and how they then put such processes into practice. The advanced practitioner cannot work alone in trying to implement changes in practice and must seek support and resources from the inter-disciplinary team. There are a number of practices that are based on practitioner preference or tradition which should be changed in line with

TABLE 8.1 Ways in which the advanced practitioner can get involved in EBP and help others to be involved

- Inter-disciplinary meetings/staff meetings;
- Clinical governance forums;
- Clinical practice committees;
- Research and audit committees/meetings;
- Project management;
- Clinical supervision;
- Teaching;
- Collaboration with higher education institutions;
- Expert role modelling.

(Whiteing, 2008)

EBP. However not all of these can be changed within a particular time-frame. The advanced practitioner should therefore work alongside colleagues to decide the areas of practice to focus on initially. Of prime importance is that the advanced practitioner must be aware of the content of the organisation's EBP/research and audit strategy to ensure that the correct procedures are followed and to avoid duplication of work amongst the team.

A change in organisational culture is often required as a first step if a change in practice is to be achieved. Often the environment or setting in which the change is to occur is a determining factor of its success (McCormack et al., 2002). As such, the advanced practitioner must inspire staff to have a shared vision rather than command and control. It is through a transformational leadership style that the advanced practitioner will achieve a change in culture and create one that is conducive to the integration of evidence into practice. Transformational leadership is an essential component of advanced practice (McGee and Castledine, 2004).

EBP and the use of Integrated Care Pathways (ICPs) (refer to the following pages) has been criticised for being too 'prescriptive' and not allowing for flexibility towards an individual's care. Whilst this could, in some instances, be true for the inexperienced practitioner looking for guidance as to the appropriate management of a patient's care episode, for the advanced practitioner it offers the opportunity to reflect on the care provided and offer alternatives for individuals and groups of patients. The community matron, for example, is well placed to look at a patient's self-management of their condition and consider these observations when planning their future care and that of others. A key element to the role of community matron is the ability to adapt a patient's package of care and pathway that allows for consideration of individual needs and preferences (Whiteing, 2008). The advanced practitioner must work both with patients to ensure that their own needs are recognised and documented within ICPs and also with staff; guiding them not to use the pathway as a protocol but to continue to look at the patients and use their own clinical judgement when planning care.

The clinically effective advanced practitioner

The advanced practitioner working as a case manager is a role that has been supported throughout the literature in providing effective care (Hickey et al., 2001; DoH, 2004; Kowalak et al., 2004; Cohen and Cesta, 2005). Indeed, many roles within the United Kingdom (UK) are adopting the role of case manager similar to that developed in the United States (US) as a way of allowing quality, outcome-focused care whilst containing costs (Cohen and Cesta, 2005). The care needs of patients are becoming more complex with an ageing population. Through the role of case manager, the advanced practitioner can meet the challenge of co-ordinating the care of patients within the increasing complexities of healthcare provision; thus practice is proactive not reactive, effective and efficient (Kowalak et al., 2004).

The Department of Health, in 2004, outlined the role of the community matron in which an advanced nurse practitioner provides case management for people with severe (three or more long term healthcare conditions) and complex health needs. Through this case management approach systematic proactive care is delivered to prevent unplanned hospital admissions and premature admission to long-term care facilities and to expedite discharge (DoH, 2004; Evans et al., 2005).

Whilst the DoH documents (2004, 2005, 2006) focus on the role of the community matron as a case manager, the content and frameworks can be applied to a range of patients being managed by the advanced practitioner in both acute and primary care environments. Indeed, in considering the three distinctive parts to clinical effectiveness outlined at the beginning of the chapter, similarities can be seen within the NHS and Social Care model for case management (DoH, 2005) whereby the case manager is required to:

- Use data to identify people who are high-end service users or at risk of unplanned hospital admission
- Re-design systems to support personalised care delivery
- Re-design and develop the workforce to meet the changed pathway of care thus reducing fragmentation
- Encourage others to use case management techniques to promote self management and minimise the burden of disease.

There is no universally agreed definition of case management. Nevertheless it should be built on a partnership that recognises patients, however vulnerable, and should be part of any decision making process (DoH, 2005). The DoH (2005, 2006) has delineated nine domains of case management practice. These can be seen in Table 8.2. These domains sit comfortably alongside the Domains and Competencies for Advanced Practice outlined by the Nursing and Midwifery Council (NMC, 2005). Indeed through meeting the competencies within the DoH's first domain and the domains competencies set out by the NMC the advanced practitioner is able to work autonomously: assessing, diagnosing, prescribing and carrying out treatments.

Through the case management model the advanced practitioner facilitates the patient's journey through the healthcare system from assessment through to discharge or referral. They should be competent in: taking medical histories; conducting physical examinations; taking responsibility for initiating and interpreting diagnostic tests; critical reasoning and diagnosis and decision making (DoH, 2005; NMC, 2005). Arrangements for consultations with specialists or specialised services and ensuring that transfers for more appropriate levels of care should be made when needed (NMC, 2005). Despite the patient's location the advanced practitioner holds responsibility for scheduling and following up test results, procedures and treatments, negotiating primary or secondary care resources and monitoring patient outcomes (Whiteing, 2008). It is more than just the patient's presenting complaint that needs to be managed by the advanced practitioner. The advanced nurse practitioner should have an appreciation of the need for prevention or treatment of health issues (Evans et al., 2005). Not all advanced practitioners will be working within a role in which they meet all of the domains and competencies for case management set out by the DoH, however the material presented is useful for workforce planners in considering the development

TABLE 8.2 Domains of case management practice

- Advanced clinical nursing practice;
- Leading complex care coordination;
- Proactively managing complex long-term conditions;
- Managing cognitive impairment and mental well-being;
- Supporting self-care, self-management and enabling independence;
- Professional practice and leadership;
- Identifying high-risk people, promoting health and preventing ill health;
- Managing care at the end of life;
- Interagency and partnership working.

(DoH, 2005, 2006)

and implementation of new advanced practice roles and the clinical effectiveness of such roles and services.

Advanced practice provides an opportunity for practitioners to redefine the traditional boundaries of practice between professions allowing continuity and co-ordination of patient care through working collaboratively with the inter-professional team. It is likely that the advanced practitioner of any professional discipline will provide a large percentage of activities for the patient. Within this context it is essential that they are able to draw upon other members of the inter-professional team and their services, as well as using critical thinking, current research and diagnostic reasoning in order to administer good quality care while ensuring efficient usage of resources (Cox, 2010a). If achieved, this will eliminate the fragmented care that is often seen as the patient moves between different departments and professionals. Patients are presenting with highly complex needs therefore it is crucial that the advanced practitioner is able to communicate effectively with other team members; striving to improve collaboration (Donagrandi and Eddy, 2000).

Following assessment of the patient and formulation of differential diagnoses a plan of care must be devised in conjunction with the other members of the inter-disciplinary team. If the management and care delivery for the patient exceeds the scope of practice of the advanced practitioner then help must be sought from more experienced colleagues. For these reasons it is essential that successful relationships with other healthcare professionals are built to ensure successful liaison and coordination of patient care. The use of the Integrated Care Pathway (ICP), discussed later in this chapter, provides an excellent platform for enhanced communication and working between different professionals.

Outside of the advanced practitioner's organisation, collaboration must also take place between acute, primary and tertiary care to ensure a smooth transition during referral or discharge. There is also a need to network with the wider health and social care network so as to appreciate wider issues (Whiteing, 2008). By having an awareness of the roles of the other healthcare team members and between different healthcare settings, the advanced practitioner can make appropriate referrals and evaluate variations from health with positive outcomes (Whiteing, 2008).

Evaluating responses to healthcare and revising practice

There is a continual pressure on healthcare providers to improve the quality of care, effectiveness and efficiency with which it is delivered. These are essential components to improving the patient's experience. In examining the quality of care delivery; the patient's response to the healthcare provided, the provider and its effectiveness must be evaluated. The advanced practitioner has a number of sources in which valuable data can be captured including patient records, policies, protocols, pathways, guidelines and standards which may provide information on the patient's responses to healthcare that is planned, has been or is being delivered and its effectiveness. The advanced practitioner should identify from patients' care plans any variances from planned pathways and work with others, including the patient, to analyse and resolve them where possible. The following section discusses a variety of ways in which patients and organisational responses to healthcare delivery can be evaluated.

Integrated care pathways (ICPs)

The ICP is being used more extensively in managing patient outcomes and care processes. ICPs are inter-disciplinary tools that outline a course of events for the treatment of patients with the same/similar conditions or undergoing similar procedures e.g., fractured neck of femur, angiogram, and appendectomy etc. Activities are placed on a timeline which depending on the place of use and condition for which the ICP has been written will vary from hourly (e.g., in an Intensive Care Unit), daily (e.g., post-operatively on a ward) or weekly (e.g., mental health setting). All activities relating to the condition/procedure are included whichever professional carries them out. Thus the ICP enables one documentation tool to be used by all professionals providing care for the patient. This facilitates enhanced communication between professionals and enables members of the team to view how the patient is progressing in other areas that may have an impact on their own activities with the patient. Importantly the ICP enables the patient to work in partnership with professionals and to review the expected goals and activities for each day that are to be achieved.

The ICP is a working document that should be regularly reviewed in line with organisational changes and research evidence that becomes available. In addition to keeping up to date with this research evidence and how it affects the ICP and subsequent patient journey, patient outcomes need to be monitored through the use of variance tracking. When a patient deviates from the planned pathway of care a variance is said to have occurred. Variances usually occur due to one or more of the following: the patient does not achieve the event (e.g., they develop a physiological problem); the practitioner omits or delays a treatment or problems are caused by the system (e.g., lack of resources, policies or procedures). Variances must be documented alongside the reasons that they have occurred and what actions have been taken. Variances should be monitored for their frequency of occurrence and their causes. Trends can be observed and practice changed as appropriate to ensure continuing clinical effectiveness of the pathway.

Case study

All patients undergoing primary joint arthroplasty surgery are cared for according to an integrated care pathway (ICP). The advanced practitioner carries out regular monitoring of variances for clinical effectiveness. An increased length of stay (LOS) of two days was found during this monitoring for those patients undergoing surgery on a Friday over those patients having surgery on any other day. Due to physiotherapy services only operating Monday to Friday it was suspected that this increase in LOS was due to inadequate physiotherapy provision.

A physiotherapy session was implemented for those patients undergoing surgery on a Friday and monitoring continued. Training was also given to nursing staff so that they could continue with rehabilitation of these patients over the weekend. As a result of the changes implemented a LOS that was equal to that of all patients undergoing arthroplasty was achieved.

Clinical audit

The importance of audit has been recognised and implemented in line with government documents (DoH, 1993a, 1994). A considerable amount of uni-disciplinary audit has been carried out over the years, however if actual benefits to patients are to occur all members of the inter-disciplinary team need to be involved in improving care and as such an audit involving all members of the inter-disciplinary team must be undertaken. The integrated care pathway discussed above provides a good platform for establishing such inter-disciplinary audits. It is through regular audits and evaluations of practice that areas for improvement and recognition of clinically effective care will be identified (Cox and Ahluwalia, 2000). For audit to be successful and have an impact it needs to be regarded as a continuous cycle rather than being a one off measurement. Audit is often referred to as a cycle or a spiral to emphasise its ongoing process.

Evaluating the patient's response to healthcare and its delivery

As of 2008, funding for hospitals has been based on a range of quality measures including: patient safety, patient experience and effectiveness of care measured through key clinical indicators (DoH, 2008a). Whilst a number of clinical measurement tools are available for measuring clinical effectiveness such as length of stay, mortality and morbidity, readmission rates, infection rates (etc); the information gleaned from them does not give any indication as to the patient's experience of their healthcare provision nor does it demonstrate whether the patient's own desired outcomes have been met. In order that healthcare can be understood and improved it is essential that the patient's perspective is sought (Hibbard, 2003; Hermann et al., 2004; Haywood, 2006; Whiteing et al., 2010/2011). It is through the use of PROMs that this data can be generated.

Patient reported outcome measures (PROMs)

Patient satisfaction is not necessarily a useful outcome measure of significant health benefit. Quality in the context of healthcare is more than patient satisfaction and whilst patient satisfaction, as an experience, is essential to measure this alone may not ensure an impact on patient outcome i.e., an improvement in health (Pennery, 2003). Nevertheless, the use of Patient Reported Outcome Measures (PROMs, 2008), are an effective instrument for discerning high quality care and areas for improvement. The advanced practitioner is in an ideal position to gather data and implement changes to healthcare delivery subsequent to PROM data collection, assessment and evaluation. It is therefore vital that they have an understanding of what PROMs are, how they are best utilised and importantly how the data gathered can be used to directly improve the patient experience (Whiteing and Cox, 2010). PROMs aim to capture and measure the patient's perspective of health status or health-related quality of life in a reliable, valid, acceptable and feasible way at a single point in time (Fitzpatrick et al., 1998; DoH, 2008b). PROMs are usually obtained through the use of a questionnaire although interviews can be utilised in some circumstances.

PROMs tools can be *generic* or *specific* (PROM, 1998). Generic tools such as the 'short form 36 version 2' (SF-36v2) (http://www.sf-36.org/) are widely applicable to patient populations and patient perceptions of their general 'generic' health status. Generic tools have the advantage of being suitable across a wide range of health problems and conditions; however this does mean that the data are not generalisable to a specific population as specific data for a disease or condition is not obtained. Specific tools allow data to be gathered on a particular health problem or population including disease/ condition specific tools, population specific tools and dimension-specific tools which focus on a particular aspect of health status e.g., cognitive functioning (Marshall et al., 2006). There are a large number of specific tools that the advanced practitioner should familiarise themselves with to enable them to choose the most appropriate tool for the proposed application.

Questionnaires used to collect PROMs can be self, interviewer or telephone-administered. Whichever method is used it is important that the user ensures that the tool is administered in the way for which it has been developed or its validity will be affected. For some patients, such as those that are unable to read or write or are housebound and unable to return a questionnaire by post, the use of a questionnaire is not the best approach to gaining information and in these circumstances a structured, semi-structured or unstructured interview or focus group can be used (Reay, 2010).

The cost of translating PROMs and re-evaluating them is high and they are not widely available in a variety of languages which can prove problematic (Whiteing and Cox, 2010). Furthermore to utilise an English language questionnaire and have a relative to translate is not acceptable as a true translation that maintains the correct meaning cannot be guaranteed (Dawson et al., 2010). Despite these problems the general evidence on PROMs is positive and the DoH is encouraging their widespread use (DoH, 2008b). PROMs have been shown to be effective in improving the nurse-patient relationship through communication (Higginson and Carr, 2001; Gilbody et al., 2003; Haywood et al., 2006) thus the use of PROMs demonstrates the advanced practitioner's contribution to Domain 1 of the Nursing and Midwifery Council's Domains and Competencies of Advanced Practice (NMC, 2005).

Activity 1

Consider how you could implement the use of PROMs within your specialty. Undertake a search for available validated tools that may be of use in gathering data in your chosen area and discuss the potential implementation of these with a colleague.

Evaluating the advanced practitioner service

In considering and ensuring clinical effectiveness the advanced practitioner has a role not only in evaluating and improving the quality of healthcare but also in evaluating his or her own practice and role within the organisation. It is essential that the advanced practitioner relate that work to outcomes for patients if they are to be valued by their colleagues, the organisation and the public (Finlay, 2000). Advanced practice roles are exciting and innovative (Furlong and Smith, 2005) however such roles need to demonstrate that outcomes are being improved and that patients' needs are being met. Thus the advanced practitioner must be able to justify their role through evaluation and outcomes research (Armstrong et al., 2002; Ball and Cox, 2003; Furlong and Smith, 2005), demonstrating how well the role is working and why and to investigate any problem areas that there may be in order that action can be taken so that they can be rectified (Walsh and Reveley, 2001; Bryant-Lukosius and DiCenso, 2004).

There are a number of ways in which the advanced practitioner and the wider team can evaluate the impact of advanced practice services including: audit, research, patient satisfaction surveys and feedback to the individual practitioner or team.

Audit trails

The role of clinical audit has been discussed previously in its contribution to ensuring clinical effectiveness. Alongside clinical audits an outcomes audit of those patients managed by the advanced practitioner will demonstrate the effectiveness of the role and resources (Griffiths, 2003). Simple records of activity, referrals, trends and outcomes can provide the advanced practitioner and the organisation with valuable data which should be used to produce activity and outcome reports to service managers as applicable. In monitoring the effectiveness and quality of the advanced practitioner service the patient's progress should be tracked once they have left their care. This may be difficult for some advanced practitioners to do, particularly those working in areas such as urgent care centres, accident and emergency and minor injury units. For the advanced practitioner working in a General Practice (GP) surgery, however, it is much easier to follow the patient up with a phone call to ensure that they are progressing well and to monitor such factors as complication rates, readmission to services and satisfaction with services.

Peer audit also offers the opportunity to formally or informally examine the quality of the advanced practice role/service in which a group of people of equal qualification/grade assess the performance of the advanced practitioner. Achieving successful audit of any type is not without difficulties and as such the advanced practitioner needs to ensure familiarity with the organisation's audit strategy, a model for use and ensure an environment that recognises the value of audit in ensuring clinical effectiveness.

Research

Nursing has tended to be involved with routine and tasks, and to be procedure driven based on opinions, tradition or habit rather than research and critical appraisal (Profetto-McGrath, 2005). The Briggs report of 1972 called for nursing to be a research-based profession and since then there have been gradual changes in education and in the uptake of a research culture. The UK government supported the Centre for Evidenced-based Nursing that is identifying ways to improve nurses' utilisation of research information (Kronenfeld et al., 2007 cited by Bickerton, 2010). Developing nurse research leaders has been part of government strategy (DoH, 2000b, 2002, 2007). This is not just applicable to nurses however and there is now an expectation that all practitioners should be aware of the research process (Cranston, 2002); particularly those working at an advanced level of practice.

The advanced practitioner should work towards gaining an understanding of a variety of research methodologies and work in a research capacity in order that not only is the service monitored and continuously improved but also to contribute to evidence-based practice as discussed at the beginning of this chapter. The key element to any study of effectiveness is the comparison between actual practice e.g., the practice by the advanced practitioner and some standard e.g., the same clinic offered by a different practitioner (Pennery, 2003). Services delivered by an advanced practitioner are often compared to those of medical practitioners, however due to the very nature of the advanced practice role; in particular the nurse as an advanced practitioner, the two services will be very different and cannot be judged by the same markers. The advanced nurse practitioner (ANP), perhaps more so than other health professionals working at an advanced level of practice, will spend much longer during a consultation due to the holistic approach taken; spending extra time on health education and addressing emotional and social elements. Whilst this may have cost implications to the organisation, in relation to time spent and productivity in ensuring clinical effectiveness, from the patient's perspective this is an important and valued aspect of service delivery.

When implementing an advanced practice service it is important that clear goals and objectives are ascertained prior to its commencement (Walsh and Reveley, 2001; Furlong and Smith, 2005; Lloyd Jones, 2005) as these are important data against which further research can be benchmarked (Walsh and Reveley, 2001). It is only through valid research evidence that opposition to advanced practice services will be overcome and continued investment in such services will continue (Walsh and Reveley, 2001; Lloyd Jones, 2005). Whilst such research activity is of importance within the advanced practitioner's organisation it is also important that the advanced practitioner has the ability to disseminate the outcomes of such investigations through written reports, conference presentations and published work that provide opportunities for others to benefit from the outcomes (McGee and Castledine, 2004).

Patient satisfaction surveys

The public's expectations of health care services are increasing and patients are far more questioning than ever before, wanting a say in how the NHS is, or should, be run (McGee and Castledine, 2004). Patient satisfaction surveys are often used and are useful in obtaining data relating to quality of services; however the data gathered can be subjective. Most patient satisfaction surveys are carried out via a questionnaire or a telephone conversation. Staniszewska and Henderson (2005) warn that surveys give an over optimistic view of the quality of care received and often do not highlight areas of poor care delivery. Patient satisfaction is dependent on the patient's individual level of expectations of services and this is based on factors such as culture and social circumstances (Walsh and Reveley, 2001); in addition patients often do not have clear reasons for their evaluations. For these reasons a follow up telephone conversation in which answers can be explored further is useful in gathering data with greater meaning.

Gathering data on patient satisfaction is extremely important in ensuring the provision of clinically effective care. Other audit measures will not obtain such data. The pitfalls of the patient satisfaction survey have been highlighted and the advanced practitioner should consider the use of PROMs (as discussed earlier) alongside such surveys. The advantage PROM tools have over routine patient satisfaction surveys that have been developed by staff is that they have been validated for their specific use and therefore data are expected to have more validity.

Feedback

Feedback from within and also external to the advanced practitioner's organisation can be helpful in developing services. This may be informal feedback through meetings or networking forums or more formal utilising the appraisal process or 360-degree feedback (Brett and Atwater, 2001). 360-degree feedback is a process whereby the advanced practitioners' own ratings as to his/her performance is compared to those ratings given anonymously by colleagues. Advanced practitioners must continue to develop their role in response to feedback received and demonstrate its effectiveness in clinical care; providing strong leadership and communicating the roles purpose, scope and education.

Activity 2

Choose an aspect of your clinical practice; consider how you might go about obtaining evidence, implementing a change and evaluating the impact of the change in your chosen area.

Maintaining competence through continuing professional development

Advanced practitioners are personally and professionally accountable for their own practice and as such must ensure their own competence to undertake the advanced practice activities to the same standard as the professional that would have traditionally undertaken them. Clinical effectiveness becomes compromised when advanced practitioners are poorly prepared for their roles and possess insufficient knowledge and skills. Several domains and competencies of advanced practice have been cited within this chapter; in working to these domains and competencies advanced practitioners will need to possess and apply an extensive repertoire of skills. To continue to be able to apply such skills, the advanced practitioner must spend a significant proportion of their time carrying out direct clinical care (McGee and Castledine, 2004). The need to maintain clinical competence through continuing professional development (CPD) and lifelong learning as well as through the review of their practice is essential (Cox, 2010b). The final part of this chapter will offer some suggestions as to ways in which the advanced practitioner can achieve this.

CPD underpins quality in the NHS, enhancing patient care (Bartle, 2000; Wood, 2004) and with a necessity to demonstrate high quality, effective and efficient interventions the importance of CPD cannot be underestimated (Clouder and Sellars, 2004; Cox, 2010b). There are two types of CPD activity that can be undertaken; those activities that focus on improving the healthcare environment e.g., conducting research, sharing of information at public forums, promotion of EBP and outcomes measurement, and those activities that focus on self-development e.g., pursuing higher education, writing for publication, staff development, reflecting on areas for development and seeking opportunities to address obtaining new skills or knowledge. Thus it can be seen that CPD can take many forms and consists of far more than attending higher education courses or just keeping 'up to date' (Whiteing, 2008). The advanced practitioner must ensure that initial training is consolidated through practice and that personal priorities for professional growth and career satisfaction are established.

Advanced practitioners must be competent in the assessment, diagnosis, treatment and care of patients whilst forming and maintaining genuine partnerships with them. To ensure clinical credibility the advanced practitioner must therefore be seen to be participating in these roles and take responsibility for their development and supervision of practice as deemed necessary (Dimond, 2003). The advanced practitioner can attend short courses and study days, shadow other members of staff within and outside of their organisation and actively participate in specialist interest groups and professional forums.

CPD activities can develop not only the individual practitioner but also the organisation and advanced practitioners now have opportunities to obtain positions in which time may be allocated to writing, undertaking research, public speaking, teaching and consulting. For the nursing profession working at an advanced level the Nursing and Midwifery Council (2005) have delineated clear Domains and Competencies of advanced practice which mirror such roles. In ensuring that practice stays up to date and therefore clinically effective the advanced practitioner may want to become involved in: teaching outside of their organisation such as at a university, writing for publication, sitting on editorial or review boards and attending and speaking at local, national and international conferences.

Clinical supervision was identified as a national initiative by the DoH in 1993 as a way of offering professional day to day support and learning in practice and assisting in ensuring safe practice (DoH,1993b). Over a decade later clinical supervision now has a role within CPD (Wood, 2004) and is supported by the NMC (2006) as a way of evaluating and improving patient care. For the advanced practitioner clinical supervision can help in the development and application of new knowledge, to manage the emotional aspects of the role and to develop standards of clinical practice (Kaur, 2003; Wood, 2004). A variety of approaches to supervision can be utilised including one-to-one supervision, group supervision and network supervision. Advanced practice roles can sometimes be isolating so the opportunity to meet with others in a clinical supervision group can be of benefit to the practitioner both in developing clinically effective practice and also as a social support mechanism. Clinical supervision is an important mechanism of support for all staff involved in care delivery (Kaur, 2003) and is not only critical to the developing advanced practitioner but also to ensuring continuing quality of the service and optimal standards of care (Clouder and Sellars, 2004).

Activity 3

Consider your own advanced practice role and how you are meeting the Domains and Competencies of advanced practice (NMC, 2005) and case management (DoH, 2005, 2006). Reflect on those domains that you are not currently meeting: consider whether this has an impact on organisational effectiveness and patient care delivery. In what ways could clinical effectiveness be improved? Do you have any specific CPD needs?

Conclusion

Measuring clinical effectiveness should not just be about the identification of potentially poor practice or performance but should be about learning from and disseminating good practice between individuals, departments and healthcare providers both locally and nationally. This chapter has looked at clinical effectiveness and ways in which the advanced practitioner can obtain and implement evidence, and evaluate the impact of changed practices. In ensuring a clinically effective service it is not enough to focus purely on organisational targets and clinical outcomes; the views of patients must also be obtained if quality healthcare is to be assured.

Those practitioners working at an advanced level hold a privileged, innovative and exciting role; one in which they have the opportunity to facilitate the patients journey through each stage of the health care system monitoring and ensuring effectiveness through a variety of means. These roles; however may be open to criticism and it is therefore important that the advanced practitioner is able to provide evidence that organisational outcomes are being achieved, improved upon and that the needs of the patients are ultimately being met.

References

Armstrong, S., Tolson, D. and West, B. (2002) Role development in acute nursing in Scotland. *Nursing Standard*, 16(17): 33–38.

Ball, C. and Cox, C. (2003) Part 1: restoring patients to health – outcomes and indicators of advanced nursing practice in adult critical care. *International Journal of Nursing Practice*, 9(6): 356–67.

Bartle, J. (2000) Clinical supervision: its place within the quality agenda. *Nursing Management*, 7(5): 30–33.

Bickerton, J. (2010) Walk-in-centre nursing: the unique nature of walk-in-centre practice, In Cox, C. and Hill, M. (Eds), 2010, *Professional Issues in Primary Care Nursing*. Oxford: Wiley-Blackwell pp. 22–38.

Brett, J. and Atwater, L. (2001) 360° feedback: accuracy, reactions and perceptions of usefulness. *Journal of Applied Psychology*, 86(5): 930–42.

Briggs, A. (1972) *Report of the committee on nursing*, London: HMSO.

Bryant-Lukosius, D. and DiCenso, A. (2004) A framework for the introduction and evaluation of advanced practice nursing roles. *Journal of Advanced Nursing*, 48: 530–40.

Burke, L., Schlenk, E., Sereika, S., Cohen, S., Happ, M. and Dorman, J. (2005) Developing competence to support evidence-based practice. *Journal of Professional Nursing*, 21(6): 358–63.

Clouder, L. and Sellars, J. (2004) Reflective practice and clinical supervision: an interprofessional perspective. *Journal of Advanced Nursing*, 46(3): 262–69.

Cohen, T. and Cesta, E. (2005) *Nursing case management from essentials to advanced practice applications*, 4th edn. St. Louis: Mosby.

Cox, C. and Ahluwalia, S. (2000) Enhancing clinical effectiveness among clinical nurse specialists. *British Journal of Nursing*, 9(16): 1064–73.

Cox, C. (2010a) *Physical Assessment for Nurses*. 2nd edn. Oxford: Wiley-Blackwell.

—— (2010b) 'APEL, APL or CPD?' International Journal of Ophthalmic Practice, 1 (1): 49–52.

Cranston, M. (2002) Clinical effectiveness and evidence-based practice. *Nursing Standard*, 16(24):39–43.

Dawson, J., Doll, H., Fitzpatrick, R., Jenkinson, C. and Carr, A. (2010) The routine use of patient reported outcome measures in healthcare settings. *British Medical Journal*, January 18, 340: c186.

DeBourgh, G. (2001) Champions for evidence-based practice: a critical role for advanced practice nurses. *Acute and Critical Care Nursing*, 12(4): 491–508.

Department of Health (1993a) *Clinical audit: meeting and improving standards in healthcare*. London: HMSO. p. 45.

—— (1993b) *A vision for the future. Report of the Chief Nursing Officer*. London: HMSO.

—— (1994) *The evolution of clinical audit*. Leeds: Department of Health.

—— (2000a) *The NHS Plan: a plan for investment, a plan for reform*. London: HMSO.

—— (2000b) *Towards a strategy for nursing research and development proposals for action*. Department of Health. Available from: http://www.dh.gov.uk/en/Publicationsandstatistics/Lettersandcirculars/Professionalletters/Chiefnursingofficerletters/DH_4004641 (accessed 14/06/2011).

—— (2002) *Nurses' use of research information in clinical decision making: A descriptive and analytical study*. Department of Health. Available from: http://www.dh.gov.uk/en/Researchanddevelopment/A-Z/Promotingimplementationresearchfindings/DH_4001837 (accessed 14/06/2011).

—— (2004) *NHS Improvement Plan 2004: Putting people at the heart of public services*. London: HMSO.

—— (2005) *Case management competenices framework for the care of people with long term conditions*. London: HMSO.

—— (2006) *Caring for people with long term conditions an education framework for community matrons and case managers*. London: HMSO.

—— (2007) *Towards a framework for post-registration nursing careers consultation document*. Department of Health. Available from: http://www.dh.gov.uk/en/Consultations/Closedconsultations/DH_079911 (accessed 14/06/2011).

—— (2008a) *High Quality Care for All. NHS Next Stage Review Final Report*. London: HMSO.

—— (2008b) *Guidance on the routine collection of Patient Reported Outcome Measures (PROMs)*. London: HMSO.

Dimond, B. (2003) *Legal and ethical issues in advanced practice*. In. McGee, P. and Castledine, G. (Eds), 2004, *Advanced Nursing Practice*, 2nd edn. Oxford: Blackwell Publishing. pp. 184–99.

Donagrandi, M. and Eddy, M. (2000) Ethics of case management: implications for advanced practice nursing. *Clinical Nurse Specialist*, 14(5): 241–49.

Evans, C., Drennan, V. and Roberts, J. (2005) Practice nurses and older people: a case management approach to care. *Journal of Advanced Nursing*, 51(4): 343–52.

Fineout-Overholt, E., Melnyk, B. and Schultz, A. (2005) Transforming health care from the inside out: Advancing evidence-based practice in the 21st century. *Journal of Professional Nursing*, 21(1): 335–44.

Finlay, T. (2000) The scope of professional practice: a literature review to determine the documents impact on nurses role. *Nursing Times Research*, 5(2): 115–25.

Fitzpatrick, R., Davey, C., Buxton, M. and Jones, D. (1998) Evaluating the patient-based outcome measures for use in clinical trials. *Health Technology Assessment*, 2(14): 1–74.

Furlong, E. and Smith, R. (2005) Advanced nursing practice; policy, education and role development. *Journal of Clinical Nursing*, 14(9): 1059–66.

Gilbody, S. M., Whitty, P. M., Grimshaw, J. M. and Thomas, R. E. (2003) Improving the detection and management of depression in primary care. *Quality and Safety in Health Care*, 12(2): 149–55.

Griffiths, M. (2003) *Evidened-based care, research and audit*. In. Palmer, D. And Kaur, S. (Eds), 2003, *Core Skills for Nurse Practitioners*. London: Whurr. pp. 57–60.

Haywood, K. (2006) Patient-reported outcome 1: measuring what matters in musculoskeletal care. *Musculoskeletal Care*, 4(4):187–203.

Haywood, K., Marshall, S. and Fitzpatrick, R. (2006) Patient participation in the consultation process: A structured review of intervention strategies. *Patient Education and Counselling*, 63(1–2): 12–23.

Hermann, R. C., Palmer, H., Leff, S., Shwartz, M., Provost, S., Chan, J., Chiv, W. T. and Lagodmos, G. (2004) Achieving consensus across diverse stakeholders on quality measures for mental healthcare. *Medical Care*, 42(12): 1246–53.

Hibbard, J. H. (2003) Engaging healthcare consumers to improve the quality of care. *Medical Care*, 41(1suppl): 161–70.

Hickey, J., Ouimette, R., Venegoni, S. (2001) *Advanced Practice Nursing*, 2nd edn. New York: Lippincott.

Higginson, I. J. and Carr, A. J. (2001) Measuring quality of life: Using quality of life measures in the clinical setting. *British Medical Journal*, 322(7297): 1297–1300.

Kaur, S. (2003) Clinical supervision. In. Palmer, D. And Kaur, S. (Eds), 2003, *Core skills for nurse practitioners*. London: Whurr. pp. 160–73.

Kowalak, J. P., Hughes, A. S. and Mills, J. E. (2004) *Best practices: A guide to excellence in nursing care*. Philadelphia: Lippincott, Williams and Wilkins.

Kronenfeld, M., Stephenson, P. L., Nail-Chiwetalu, B., Tweed, E. M., Sauers, E. L., McLeod, T. C., Guo, R., Trahan, H., Alpi, K. M., Hill, B., Sherwill-Navarro, P., Allen, M. P., Stephenson, P. L., Hartman, L. M., Burnham, J., Fell, D., Pavlick, R., MacNaughton, E. W. and Ratner, N. B. (2007) cited in Bickerton, J. (2010) Use of theory and research to inform practice. In. Cox, C. and Hill, M. (Eds), 2010, *Professional issues in primary care nursing*. Oxford: Wiley-Blackwell. p. 187.

Levin, R. and Feldman, H. (2006) *Teaching Evidenced Based Practice in Nursing: A Guide for Academic and Clinical Settings*. New York: Springer.

Lloyd Jones, M. (2005) Role development and effective practice in specialist and advanced practice roles in acute hospital settings: systematic review and meta-synthesis. *Journal of Advanced Nursing*, 49(2): 191–209.

Marshall, S., Haywood, K. and Fitzpatrick, R. (2006) Impact of patient-reported outcome measures on routine practice: a structured review. *Journal of Evaluation in Clinical Practice*, 12(5): 559–68.

McCormack, B., Kitson, A., Harvey, G., Rycroft-Malone, J., Titchen, A. and Seers, K. (2002) Getting evidence into practice: the meaning of context. *Journal of Advanced Nursing*, 38(1): 94–104.

McGee, P. and Castledine, G. (2004) Future directions in advanced nursing practice in the UK. In. McGee, P. and Castledine, G. (Eds.), (2004) *Advanced Nursing Practice*, 2nd edn. Oxford: Blackwell. pp. 225–37.

Munro, N. (2004) Evidence-based assessment: no more pride or prejudice. *Acute and Critical Care Nursing*, 15: 501–5.

NHS Executive (1996) *Promoting Clinical Effectiveness: A Framework for Action in and Through the NHS*. Leeds: Department of Health.

Nursing and Midwifery Council (2005) *Annex 1 Domains of Practice and Competencies, NMC Consultation on a Proposed Framework for Post-registration Nursing*. London: NMC.

—— (2006) *Clinical supervision*. London: NMC.

Patient Reported Outcome Measurement (2008) Instrument Types. Available from: http://phi.uhce.ox.ac.uk/inst_types.php (accessed 14/06/2011)

Pennery, E. (2003) Effectiveness and evaluation of the nurse-led clinic. In. Hatchet, R. (Ed), 2003, *Nurse led clinics practice issues*. London: Routledge. pp. 69–86.

Profetto-McGrath, J. (2005) Critical thinking and evidence-based practice. *Journal of Professional Nursing*, 21(6): 364–71.

Reay, N. (2010) How to measure patient experience and outcomes to demonstrate quality in care. *Nursing Times*, 106(7): 12–14.

Rycroft-Malone, J., Harvey, G., Kitson, A., McCormack, B., Seers, K. and Titchen, A. (2002) Getting evidence into practice: ingredients for change. *Nursing Standard*, 16(37):38–43.

SF 36 (2010) *Short Form 36 Health Survey*. http://www.sf-36.org (accessed 14/06/2011)

Staniszewska, A. and Henderson, A. (2005) Patients' evaluations of the quality of care: influencing factors and the importance of engagement. *Journal of Advanced Nursing*, 49(5): 530–37.

Walsh, M. and Reveley, S. (2001) Evaluating the nurse practitioner role in hospital. In. Reveley, S. Walsh, M. and Crumbie, A. (Eds) 2001, *Nurse practitioners developing the role in hospital settings*. Oxford: Butterworth Heinemann. pp. 130–43.

Whiteing, N. L. (2008) Domain 7: Monitoring and ensuring the quality of health care practice. In. Hinchliff, S. and Rogers, R. (Eds.), 2008, *Competencies for advanced nursing practice*. London: Hodder Arnold. pp. 192–219.

Whiteing, N. and Cox, C. (2010) Using Patient Reported Outcome Measures to improve patient care. *Journal of Gastrointestinal Nursing*, 8(5): 16–19

Whiteing, N., Cox, C. and Bentley, P. (2010/2011) Patient Reported Outcome Measures in Ophthalmology, *International Journal of Ophthalmic Practice*, 1(2): 28–34, December/January

Wood, J. (2004) Clinical supervision. *British Journal of Perioperative Nursing*, 14(4): 151–56.

Chapter 9   **Influencing Others**

Kathryn Waddington

Introduction

Dale Carnegie's (1937/2006) classic bestseller *How to Win Friends and Influence People* has sold over 15 million copies, indicating that there is an enduring interest in the concept of influence. The ability to influence others is an important aspect of leadership and advanced practice, closely linked with associated concepts of followership, power and political awareness (Ball and Cox, 2004; Northouse, 2010). In an increasingly competitive health economy, healthcare professionals and managers now need to become much more business-minded. The ability to understand and use power and influence is crucial. The current business of healthcare and public sector reform demands that practitioners must continue to provide ever-improving reliable and high quality services, whilst simultaneously reconfiguring and dismantling these same services (Pederson and Hartley, 2008). At work, and outside work, people are faced with the task of influencing others to do something which they may not want to do – something which requires them to change, or to behave in different ways. The ability to influence others therefore is a transferable skill and an important aspect of continuing personal and professional development.

This chapter draws upon theoretical perspectives and research from social and organisational psychology, public sector management and nursing, inter-woven and applied to the emerging interdisciplinary field of interprofessional collaborative practice (Suter and Deutschlander, 2010; Waddington, 2010a). In order to fully engage with the material and activities to enhance learning available in this chapter it is recommended that you use approaches to critical reflection which address the issues and dynamics of power and powerless-ness (Bishop, 2009; Brookfield, 2009; Fook and Gardner, 2007). These are developed in more depth later in this chapter.

Learning Outcomes

At the conclusion of this chapter you will be able to:

- Demonstrate awareness of contemporary perspectives and theories of leadership and followership
- Identify the types of power within and between individuals, professions and healthcare systems
- Understand the need to use different influencing styles and tactics within a wider context of developing political awareness
- Appreciate the tensions between value-based inter/professional practice and economically focussed business approaches
- Critically reflect upon your own influencing and interpersonal skills, and how they impact upon advanced practice and the delivery of reconfigured services.

The chapter is organised as follows. First the concepts of social influence and interprofessional collaborative practiced are introduced, followed by a more detailed exploration of leadership, followership, power and politics. Then there is a selection of learning activities and case study material designed to develop influencing skills by advancing your self awareness, knowledge and skills of critical reflection.

Background

There is evidence that poor interprofessional communication and ineffective collaboration results in avoidable deaths and causes serious harm to patients, communities and society (Laming, 2009; Suter and Deutschlander, 2010). The World Health Organization (WHO, 2010) has predicted a global healthcare workforce crisis across all health provider groups. The need to resolve these issues is urgent, as is an understanding of the ways that healthcare professionals interact and influence each other in the *shared* endeavour of advancing practice. It is pertinent at this point to clarify key terms and underlying concepts relating to social influence and interprofessional collaboration which provide the background and context for application of theoretical and practical materials which follow later in the chapter.

Social influence

The term influence is defined as 'the act, power, or capacity of causing or producing an effect in somebody or something, *especially* in indirect or intangible ways' (*The New Penguin English Dictionary*). It comes from the Latin *influere*, meaning to flow, indicating that influence is not static; rather it is a dynamic process. In psychological terms, social influence is broadly defined as the process whereby people directly or indirectly influence the thoughts, feelings and attitudes of others, and is linked to persuasion, conformity and attitude change (Pratkanis, 2007). It is also relevant however to consider what influencing is *not*; it is not bullying, coercing, forcing, manipulating or dictating. Social influence is also closely associated with social capital, defined as '*investment in social relations with expected returns*' (Stevenson and Radin, 2009:19; italics in original). Social capital is an important resource that exists in networks and interprofessional relationships, and is possessed by individual practitioners, collectively in teams and units, and is an important aspect of collaborative practice (Forbes, 2009).

Interprofessional collaboration

In the U.K. over the last 20 years partnership working and inter-agency collaboration have been part of the government rhetoric and language of professional and interprofessional practice. European Union (EU) and World Health Organisation (WHO) European Region policy mandate the need for collaborative interagency, interprofessional and inter-sectoral practice (Waddington, 2010a). It is important to find and use shared language and frameworks to describe and understand interprofessional practice, yet the picture is confusing. Butt et al. (2008) note that the terms collaboration, partnership teamwork, interdisciplinary and interprofessional are used interchangeably. However broad conceptual distinctions between interprofessional, interagency, multi-agency and partnership approaches have been also been discerned (Curran, 2007; Stepney and Callwood, 2006). Waddington (2010a:211) notes that an interprofessional approach involves:

> Professionals from different disciplinary backgrounds (e.g., nursing, social work, medicine, physiotherapy) working together more effectively, often in teams, to improve the quality of care provided to individuals, families and communities.
>
> Interprofessional collaboration therefore is the *process* through which different professional groups work together, and sharing information, learning and knowledge to positively impact on healthcare (Zwarenstein et al., 2009). However this is not necessarily an easy process and an understanding of power, politics and leadership is necessary to work with the complex dynamics of influencing others in an interprofessional arena.
> (Waddington, 2010a:211)

Key information addressing learning outcomes

Influencing is about moving people in a different direction, but without forcing, bullying or coercion and is also about knowing and understanding yourself, and the effect you have on other people. According to Dent and Brent (2006), being an effective influencer requires patience and a willingness to practise new skills, leading to enhanced decision making, better participation and higher motivation. This section addresses key aspects of leadership, follower-ship, power and politics in order to help you critically reflect upon your own influencing style and skills.

Leadership, leading and following

Leadership is a complex and ambiguous topic, with multiple definitions and shifting perspectives all of which, to some extent, include elements of persuasion and influencing (Drath et al., 2008). The notion of 'leadership as influence' is based on the assumption that a leader is capable of generating more influence than followers. For example Northouse (2010: 3) defines leadership as 'a process whereby an individual influences a group of individuals to achieve a common goal'. However there is an important distinction to be made between leadership as an influencing process, and the relationship between leading and following. Leaders need followers, but followers are not necessarily passive recipients of leaders' influence and practitioners are increasingly working in contexts where this asymmetrical leader/follower relationship is absent. Such contexts include interprofessional teams where clinicians, who might all be leaders in their own field of professional practice, are working together in a partnership process of managing and promoting health. In these contexts leadership is being reconstructed. It is a relational and co-constructed phenomenon which acknowledges the *mutual influences* of leaders and the people around them. This approach to leadership aligns with a collaborative interprofessional practice approach, and allows for the inclusion of patients/service users and communities on a more equal basis.

Shifting to this reconstructed, collaborative approach to leadership calls for a shift in thinking, reframing leadership in terms of outcomes. In this sense, leadership is more about producing agreement on *direction*, creating a framework for *alignment*, and a sense of *commitment* to the collective endeavour (Drath et al., 2008). A collaborative approach also requires a rethinking of the influence that particular professions and clinicians hold, and how power is distributed and shared.

Power

Power is a complex concept, often viewed negatively in terms of its potential to bully or coerce. The processes of power are overt or covert and manifest in many different guises like gossip and organisational 'status symbols' such as office furnishings and desk size. Power is often unequally distributed in organisations, and individuals and groups may be disadvantaged on the basis of class, race, gender or profession. The ways in which power is gained, used, legitimised, concealed and abused is frequently the topic of daily conversations, as well as being the subject of theoretical analysis and research (Clegg et al., 2006; Fineman et al., 2010; Waddington and Michelson, 2011).

Any theoretical discussion of power would be incomplete without acknowledgement of the influence of French philosopher Michel Foucault. His thesis is that it is impossible to separate power from knowledge, that they are not neutral concepts, and that all knowledge is dangerous (Foucault, 1982). Power is not a 'thing' or a 'capacity' but is: (i) a network of relations that are localized, dispersed, diffused and typically disguised through a social system; (ii) productive of particular types of knowledge and social order; and (iii) operating at the most micro levels of social relations. Foucault's work is extensive and complex, and word limits means that it cannot be addressed in detail here, but it is important for two reasons. Firstly, health and medicine significantly influenced his thinking and theorising about knowledge and power (Bishop, 2009). Secondly, because questions about the power relationships which allow, or promote, one set of practices to be considered more effective than others are essential to critical (as opposed to uncritical) reflection and interprofessional collaborative practice.

Power can be thought of as a *capacity to influence*, and distinguished from *influence* which is the actual use of power by specific behaviour(s), which changes other people's actions thoughts or feelings (Klocke, 2009). Power as capacity to influence can be seen in terms of French and Raven's (1959) now classic social psychology theory of social power. This theory rests on the assumption that influence involves a relationship between at least two individuals, initially based upon five types of power: (i) reward; (ii) coercive; (iii) position; (iv) legitimate; and (v) referent, but which can now be expanded to include power relating to information and relationships with influential others, in other words social capital as outlined above. These different types of power are illustrated in Table 9.1.

Power can be further differentiated into *situational* sources, such as position in the team/organisation and *personal* sources, for example individual attributes such as integrity and interpersonal skills. There are also cultural differentiations

TABLE 9.1 Types of Power

Type of power	Assumptions about person influencing
Reward	Based on perception that positive rewards can be given and/or negative outcomes can be removed.
Coercive	Based on perception that they can administer penalties/sanctions to those who do not comply.
Referent	Power arises from the individual's personal characteristics and traits which are respected and admired.
Legitimate	Possession of authority as a consequence of their role/position in the organisation with associated rights to demand compliance in others.
Expert	Based on possession of distinctive knowledge, skills, expertise relevant to the task and context.
Information	Based upon access to and/or control over information.
Connection	Derived from relationships and networks with other powerful people.

and differences in the perceptions and acceptance of power in institutions (Hofstede, 1980). Hofstede's seminal text on cross-cultural differences in organisations, *Culture's Consequences: International Differences in Work-Related Values* outlines a cultural value framework which includes the dimension of 'power distance', defined as: 'the extent to which a society *accepts* the fact that power in institutions and organizations is distributed unequally' (Hofstede, 1980:45, emphasis added). It is also the extent to which subordinates are not expected to express disagreement with their supervisors, and supervisors are not expected to consult with their subordinates in the decision-making process. The healthcare workforce is diverse and hierarchical, and in recent years the NHS and other health sector employers have been active in recruiting health professionals internationally (Buchan et al., 2005). There are therefore cross-cultural differences with regard to the way that individual practitioners may accept and expect unequal distribution of power which need to be understood and managed sensitively.

There is also another distinction between the *formal* and *informal* constraints of power (Fineman et al., 2010). Formal power in healthcare is found within systems, managerial hierarchies and professions, particularly medicine, which may either facilitate or hinder other professionals' ability to practice effectively. Paynton's (2008) research illustrates the tactics that hospital-based nurses in the U.S. used to 'work-around' what were perceived as inappropriate decisions made by physicians, in order to advocate on behalf of their patients. In this study the 'doctor-nurse' game (Stein 1967, cited in Paynton, 2008), in which nurses use communication strategies to make their suggestions appear as if they were the doctors' ideas was one of the tactics adopted. Yet using informal power strategies such as this are detrimental to achieving enhanced professional autonomy and recognition because nurses are sacrificing their own formal power to fulfil an advanced practice role.

Contemporary interprofessional practice requires *all* healthcare professionals to collaborate on a higher level of mutual respect and trust. However as Reeves et al. (2008:2) comment 'the web of structural factors such as professional power and gender that must be modified to find this new level of collaboration is not going to make this an easy path.' Nevertheless, this collaborative path can be made easier by having a deeper understanding of the political context of practice, and the ability to lead, follow and manage with political awareness.

Politics

Organisational/professional politics have traditionally held connotations of disreputable self-interested individual behaviour, 'protecting your turf' and 'watching your back', involving formation of alliances, plots and dirty tricks. As Fineman et al. (2010:424) note:

> Organizations with proclaimed strong **ethical** systems such as hospitals and churches are, ironically, notorious for the robustness of their organizational politics. Indeed, one observer suggests that the more people believe that what they are doing is for the good of others, the dirtier tricks they are prepared to resort to in order to get their way.
>
> Fineman et al. (2010:424, emphasis in original)

The understanding of organisational politics and the development of political awareness is becoming an increasingly important managerial and leadership skill (Hartley et al., 2007).

Ball and Cox's (2004:11) research into advanced nursing practice in adult critical care also found that political awareness is central to facilitating 'legitimate influence', the purpose of which is to enhance patient stay and improve patient outcome. With regard to advanced clinical practice, political awareness entails the manipulation of various bureaucratic systems in order to expedite patient movement through various departments. This was demonstrated in Ball and Cox's (2004:18) study by having 'a sense of the game plan' and the need not to push things too far, too quickly.

Politics is being reconceptualised and understood using different terms such as partnership working, influencing and communication skills. Hartley et al.'s (2007) political skills framework, based upon research across an extensive senior management population identified five interconnected dimensions of political skill: (i) personal skills; (ii) interpersonal skills; (iii) reading people and situations; (iv) building alignment and alliances; and (v) strategic direction and planning. Personal and interpersonal skills form the foundations upon which trust and the understanding of the needs and interests of other individuals and organisations are built. The ability to read people and situations is about the ability to interpret people's motives, agendas and interests in different situations. Skills of alliance building across different professional perspectives are crucial for setting shared agendas and strategic direction. Table 9.2 outlines Hartley et al's (2007:7) political skills framework illuminated by data from Ball and Cox's (2004) skills of political awareness as described by advanced nurse practitioners.

TABLE 9.2 Dimensions of Political Skills and Awareness in Advanced Practice

Dimensions of political skills	Political awareness in advanced practice
Strategic direction and scanning	... (being) really involved in some strategic management and planning long-term ...
Building alignment and alliances	... I guess that my knowledge base comes a lot from just networking with other people and finding out what is available but now that I know that I can expedite people.... through the department ...
Reading people and situations	... didn't make me very popular but I didn't have to worry about it. I wasn't popular; nobody knew who I was anyway. So it was a perfect time to disrupt the system.
Interpersonal skills	I'm always very mindful of the messages that I give out, you know, when I work clinically, role modelling, in discussions, in meetings, whatever, I'm very mindful about that all the time ...
Personal skills	... if you're one day saying 'Well, let's do things a bit different' then it has a very powerful effect on people so that you've got to be very clear in your own mind about values and beliefs, what you think is important.

(based on Ball and Cox, 2004; Hartley et al., 2007)

Political skills and awareness form part of a model of influencing summarised in Table 9.3, which links the key information from this section with the activities to enhance learning which follow.

TABLE 9.3 A Model of Influencing

Step 1:	Understanding and being aware of the influencing environment – e.g., organisational culture and related behaviours that are sanctioned, and those which are not acceptable;
Step 2:	Self awareness of interpersonal skills and preferred influencing styles – e.g., listening, questioning and probing, body language, 'push' and 'pull' styles, 'hard' and 'soft' tactics;
Step 3:	Identifying the needs/wants of all parties being influenced, their power bases and preferences;
Step 4:	Reviewing – e.g., what is known about the influencing environment/context, planning next actions;
Step 5:	Identifying and using tools/techniques or approaches to influencing others, based upon the situation, people and issues involved;
Step 6:	Critically reflecting upon the processes of influencing, the outcomes for all involved, and the way that power was manifest and used.

(based on Dent and Brent, 2006)

Activities to enhance learning

These activities have been designed to facilitate and enhance your learning. They can be used alone or with colleagues, and it is also recommended that you make use of journals and/or other tools for critical reflection (Bolton, 2010; Fook and Gardner, 2007). Critical reflection journals can be used by individual practitioners, and also by interprofessional teams, for example to note significant incidents that relate to policy implementation and service reconfiguration over a period of time.

Critical reflection

The learning activities are guided by the principles of critical reflection, summarised by Fook and Gardner (2007:16) as encompassing the following attributes:

- Reflection is deeper than popular notions of 'thinking'
- Critical reflection is based on an understanding of the individual in social contexts and links between individual and society

- Critical reflection is both a *theory* and a *practice*
- Critical reflection links changed awareness with changed action.

Critical reflection also calls into question the power relationships that allow or promote one set of practices or professional values over another:

> For reflection to be considered critical it must have as its explicit focus uncovering, and challenging, the power dynamics that frame practice and uncovering and challenging hegemonic assumptions (those assumptions we embrace as being in our best interests when in fact they are working against us).
>
> (Brookfield, 2009:293)

In other words do not be afraid to ask yourself: *What is really going on here?* There are also other questions (Refer to Waddington, 2010b:238) that you can ask yourself – and colleagues – in order to access and surface deeper organisational patterns and dynamics of power. For example:

- What behaviours are rewarded by the organisation and what typical patterns of behaviour do you notice at meetings?
- What stories and gossip are circulating in the 'unmanaged spaces', for example tales of the unexpected heroes, villains and fools?
- What/who would be included in the 'unofficial induction programme'?
- What are the 'organisational secrets' – the things that most people know, but which cannot be talked about openly? Why are these issues not confronted?

The learning activities which follow are not prescriptive, you may well have come across some of them before, and it is up to you to decide how best to use them. For instance you may choose to work through these exercises sequentially, dip in and out, or return to them later when you have had time to think and reflect. What *is* important is that you think carefully and critically about your own history, experience and approach to influencing – and being influenced by – others. You may want to do them more than once, or make a commitment to review your influencing skills on a regular basis, for example in preparation for appraisal, in preparation for a job application or when updating your CV. Your developing self awareness, critical reflection skills and learning about influencing can also be utilised in other leadership and management development activities such as coaching and/or mentoring.

Activity 1: Critical Incident Analysis

Identify a situation/incident in which you needed or wanted to influence others. Say why it was significant, and describe the context/background/other people involved.

Now identify anything in the situation/incident that you found particularly difficult about influencing others; use the suggested questions below for critical reflection and to write a reflective journal entry.

Questions to promote critical reflection:

*   What was *really* going on there?
*   What were the underlying issues?
*   What types of power were available to me? (Refer to Table 1 above)
*   Did I use my power effectively/appropriately?
*   Were any voices/views not being heard?
*   How did I come across to other people?
*   What might other people have said about me/the incident afterwards?
*   What is my next action?

Having completed this activity you should have been able to identify your sources of power, which can be thought of as *energy*, and you may also want to think literally and metaphorically about your sources of power as energy. For example is it renewable and sustainable like solar power? Does it have any potential damaging by products like nuclear power? Is it reliant on fossil fuels which will run out at some point in the future?

Activity 2: Push and Pull Influencing Styles

This activity requires you to think critically about your own influencing style and interpersonal skills. After completing Activity 1 you should have identified your sources of power, which can be thought of as *energy* used for pushing and pulling.

continued . . .

Activity 2: Push and Pull Influencing Styles ... *continued*

Push Pull

- Work to your own agenda
- Focus on your needs
- State your motives or reasoning
- Make proposals or suggest ideas
- Say how you feel
- Find out about their agenda
- Focus on their needs
- Find out their motivations or reasoning
- Seek out other proposals or ideas
- Find out how they feel.

If you only ever push you may be seen as imposing but self-centred, focussing only on yourself/your service rather than others; if you only ever pull you may be seen as interested but unclear as to your own needs and goals. When working interprofessionally, every situation calls for an assessment of the balance between push and pull energies needed to achieve shared goals.

To develop self awareness of your influencing style, ask yourself the following questions:

- Why do people do what I want them to do?
- What is it about me that wins people over?
- What is it that that I do which gets other people's cooperation?
- What connections do I have that other people value?
- Is there anything about my approach which sways people?

It may be helpful to enlist the help of a friend or trusted colleague to act as a 'critical companion' who can give you feedback on your answers. Finding out why other people think you are – or are not – powerful or influential can be very illuminating.

Having identified your own sources of power and how they can be used, it is now pertinent to look more widely at power within relational systems and begin to map the patterns of influence around you and your team/service.

Activity 3: Influence Mapping

Influence mapping is a way of identifying the individuals and groups who hold power, and is a way of assessing their position and motives. It is similar to Lewin's Force Field Analysis, and the approach adopted here is that of Practice Genograms which can be used to understand systems and visualize complex organisational relationships.

For the purpose of this activity 'practice' can be addressed at a number of different levels of analysis – e.g., team, unit, ward, agency or organisational. The technique is based upon the principles used in family genograms, but you do not need to be familiar with working with families in order to use this approach to influence mapping.

You will need a large piece of paper, different coloured pens in order to make a visual representation of the following:

*   Key members and their roles;
*   Demographics – e.g., age, gender, length of time in role;
*   Hierarchies, coalitions and boundaries;
*   Existing relationships and networks;
*   Stage in the 'life cycle' – e.g., emergent/mature/declining;
*   Important recent events/history;
*   Implicit and explicit belief systems;
*   Powerful people – e.g., overt/covert, formal/informal sources of power;
*   Communication styles/approach.

Visually, a Practice Genogram may be similar to an organisational chart, but with the addition of elements that identify the informal, emotional and relational patterns within the structure.

This is a powerful tool for identifying key decision-makers, opinion leaders, enablers and saboteurs, and is particularly valuable in interprofessional collaborative projects and change management.

Case Studies – Influencing Tactics

The aim of the following two short case studies is to illustrate how 'hard' and 'soft' influence tactics can impact upon teamwork and perceptions. Hard influence tactics include pressure, assertiveness, forming coalitions and blocking; soft influence tactics include rational persuasion, inspirational appeals and consultation (Klocke, 2009).

Case study 1 – Mo

Mo is an ambitious manager with plans to undertake an MBA (Masters in Business Administration) in healthcare management, and has aspirations to work in a strategic role at Board or Directorate level. Mo has recently been promoted to lead a team working on a high profile service transformation project. This project is seen as key to implementing the nursing strategy, as well as enabling the hospital to deliver their business agenda. In project meetings Mo produces management information, statistics and reports, which support a quick implementation of the reconfigured service, but has a tendency to ignore or interrupt dissenting views. Mo is very clear about what needs to be done and is not afraid to use pressure and sanctions, but there is a perception in the team of 'divide and rule' tactics. Individual members of the team also disagree amongst themselves as to whether Mo's approach represents a tough management approach needed for tough times, or bullying and harassment.

Case study 2 – Fran

Fran is also ambitious with plans to undertake PhD (Doctoral) studies and become a nurse consultant. Fran has recently been appointed into an advanced nurse practitioner (ANP) post. The ANP job description includes specific responsibility for the development and implementation of a strategy for the management of long term conditions within a community adult nursing team. In meetings Fran ensures that information is gathered from all practitioners, encouraging everyone to express their views and draw upon their experience. Fran is also involving patients and carers, reviewing the literature, and taking time to develop a strategy which integrates all these perspectives. Fran's boss is under pressure from the Director of Nursing to get the strategy signed off and implemented, and is beginning to question whether Fran was the right person for the job. The doctors are expressing frustration over still having to see patients they were expecting to be able refer to nurse practitioners.

Activity 4: Reflecting on the Case Studies

The following questions are just a start. You may also have other questions as a result of reading, thinking and engaging in learning activities in this chapter:

- What other tactics and approaches could Mo and Fran have used in each case study?
- What tactics and approaches would you adopt if you were in similar situations, either as the person influencing, or the person being influenced?
- How can tensions between value-based professional practice and the 'business of healthcare' be addressed?
- How can practitioners practise critical reflection in times of financial austerity?
- How can teams harness and effectively use their collective interprofessional power and influence?

Conclusion

The ability to influence and communicate effectively is an essential aspect of advanced practice, and crucial to the delivery of effective services which are under threat or subject to reconfiguration and change. This chapter should have helped you to think about and critically reflect upon the ways in which you influence people, the approaches you use and the importance of leading, managing and practising with political awareness. By working through the learning activities you should now be aware that influencing other people is often more about changing *your* attitudes and behaviour than it is about changing theirs. Taking time to think about your own approach, interpersonal and communication skills and getting feedback from others can help you to become a more effective influencer. Careful consideration and challenging of the complex, and often hidden, aspects of power in professional practice are fundamental to the development of enabling – rather than disabling – interprofessional collaborative cultures.

The final learning activity *in this chapter* then is about identifying key action points and areas for future development of your influencing skills and knowledge. However your day-to-day work experience and conversations with colleagues should also provide a rich source of material for further learning, as will the additional internet-based resources that are found at the end of the chapter.

Activity 5: Next Steps

Look back over the material contained in this chapter and consider the following:

- What key action points can you identify to improve your influencing skills – i.e., what are the things you will start doing, keep doing or stop doing?
- Have you identified any gaps in your knowledge and/or skills?
- If so how might any further training or development help – e.g., further reading, attending training courses, coaching, mentoring, work shadowing etc.
- How will you use your sources of power and influencing skills to lead advanced practice in your area of work?
- How will you enable others to develop their own influencing skills and practice?

References

Ball, C. and Cox, C. L. (2004) Part two: The core components of legitimate influence and the conditions that constrain or facilitate advanced nursing practice in adult critical care, *International Journal of Nursing Practice*, 13(10): 10–20.

Bishop, J. P. (2009) Revisiting Foucault, *The Journal of Medicine and Philosophy*, 34(4): 323–27.

Bolton, G. E. J. (2010) *Reflective Practice: Writing and Professional Development*, 3rd Ed. London: Sage.

Brookfield, S. (2009) The concept of critical reflection: Promises and contradictions, *European Journal of Social Work*, 12(3): 293–304.

Buchan, J., Jobanputra, R., Gough, P. and Hutt, R. (2005) *Internationally Recruited Nurses in London*. London: Kings Fund.

Butt, G., Markle-Reid, M. and Browne, G. (2008) Interprofessional partnerships in chronic illness care: a conceptual model for measuring partnership effectiveness. *International Journal of Integrated Care*, 8. Available at: http://www.ijic.org/ (accessed 01/08/2010).

Carnegie, D. (1937/2006) *How to Win Friends and Influence People*. New York: Pocket Books.

Clegg, S. R., Courpasson, D. and Phillips, N. (2006) *Power and Organizations*. London: Sage.

Curran, V. (2007) *Collaborative Care*. Ottawa: Health Canada Publications.

Dent, F. and Brent, M. (2006) *Influencing: Skills and Techniques for Business Success*. Basingstoke: Palgrave Macmillan.

Drath, W. H., McCauley, C. D., Palus, C. J., Van Velsor, E., O'Connor, P. M. G. and McGuire, J. B. (2008) Direction, alignment, commitment: Toward a more integrative ontology of leadership, *The Leadership Quarterly*, 19, 635–53.

Fineman, S., Gabriel, Y. and Sims, D. (2010) *Organizing and Organizations*, 4th Ed. London: Sage.

Fook, J. and Gardner, F. (2007) *Practising Critical Reflection: A Resource Handbook*. Maidenhead: Open University Press/McGraw Hill.

Forbes, J. (2009) Redesigning children's services: Mapping interprofessional social capital, *Journal of Research in Special Educational Needs*, 9(2): 122–32.

Foucault, M. (1982) The subject and power, pp. 208–26 in H. Dryfus and P. Rabinow (Eds), *Michel Foucault: Beyond Structuralism and Hermeneutics*. London: Harvester Wheatsheaf.

French, J. R. P. Jr. and Raven, B. H. (1959) The bases of social power, pp. 105–67 in D. Cartwright (ed.), *Studies in Social Power*. Ann Arbour: University of Michigan Press.

Hartley, J., Fletcher, C., Wilton, P., Woodman, P. and Ungemach, C. (2007) *Leading with Political Awareness: developing leaders' skills to manage the political dimension across all sectors*. London: Chartered Management Institute.

Hofstede, G. (1980) *Culture's Consequences: International Differences in Work-Related Values*. Newbury Park, CA: Sage.

Klocke, U. (2009) I am the best: Effects of influence tactics and power bases on powerholders' self-evaluation and target evaluation, *Group Processes & Intergroup Relations*, 12(5): 619–37.

Laming, The Lord (2009) *The Protection of Children in England: A Progress Report*. London: The Stationary Office. Available at: http://publications.education.gov.uk/eOrderingDownload/HC-330.pdf (accessed 14/06/2011)

The New Penguin English Dictionary (2000), London: Penguin Books Ltd.

Northouse, P. G. (2010) *Leadership: Theory and Practice* 4th Ed. Thousand Oaks CA: Sage.

Paynton, S. T. (2008) The informal power of nurses for promoting patient care, *The Online Journal of Issues in Nursing*, Vol. 14, No. 1. Available from: http://www.nursingworld.org/MainMenuCategories/ANAMarketplace/ANAPeriodicals/OJIN/TableofContents/vol142009/No1Jan09/ArticlePreviousTopic/InformalPowerofNurses.aspx (accessed 14/06/2011).

Pederson, D. and Hartley, J. (2008) The changing context of public leadership and management: Implications for roles and dynamics, *International Journal of Public Sector Management*, 21(4): 327–39.

Pratkanis, A. R. (2007) *The Science of Social Influence: Advances and future progress*. Hove: The Psychology Press.

Reeves, S., Nelson, S. and Zwarenstein, M. (2008) The doctor–nurse game in the age of interprofessional care: A view from Canada, *Nursing Inquiry*,18(1): 1–2.

Stein, L. I. (1967) 'The doctor-nurse game', *Archives of General Psychiatry*, 16(6): 699–703.

Stepney, P. and Callwood, I. (2006) *Collaborative working in health and social care: a review of the literature*. Wolverhampton: University of Wolverhampton. Available from: http://wlv.openrepository.com/wlv (accessed 14/06/2011)

Stevenson, W. B. and Radin, R. F. (2009) Social capital and social influence on the board of directors, Journal *of Management Studies*, 46(1): 16–44.

Suter, E. and Deutschlander, S. (2010) *Can Interprofessional Collaboration Provide Health Human Resources Solutions? A knowledge synthesis*. Available from: http://www.hrhresourcecenter.org/node/3052 (accessed 14/06/2011)

Waddington, K. (2010a) Collaboration and working with the multidisciplinary team and agencies, pp. 209–25 in C. Cox and M. Hill (eds.) *Professional Issues in Primary Care Nursing*. Oxford: Wiley Blackwell.

—— (2010b) Leadership and organisational decision making: the nurse's role in policy and practice, pp. 226–42 in C. Cox & M. Hill (eds.) *Professional Issues in Primary Care Nursing*. Oxford: Wiley Blackwell.

Waddington, K. and Michelson, G. (2011) *Gossip and Organizations*. London: Routledge.

World Health Organization (WHO) (2010) *Framework for Action on Interprofessional Education and Collaborative Practice*. Available at: http://www.who.int/hrh/resources/framework_action/en/index.html (accessed 14/06/2011).

Zwarenstein, M., Goldman, J. and Reeves, S. (2009) Interprofessional collaboration: effects of practice-based interventions on professional practice and healthcare outcomes. *Cochrane Database of Systematic Reviews*, Issue 3. Art. No.: CD000072. DOI: 10.1002/14651858.CD000072.pub2.

Internet-based Resources

http://mcgraw-hill.co.uk/openup/fook&gardner/

This website accompanies Fook and Gardner's (2007) *Practising Critical Reflection: A Resource Handbook* and contains a variety of helpful resources to support critical reflective practice, including examples of critical incident analysis, additional articles and reading materials and sample material for workshop preparation.

http://my-ecoach.com/

This is an online learning community built on a coaching platform which offers collaboration, communication, curriculum, resources, and publishing tools, such as the *Developing Personal Skills: Influencing Styles Push and Pull Questionnaire*.

http://www.cln.nhs.uk/

This is the website for the *Clinical Leaders Network* a national, professional leadership network for clinicians in England, bringing together a broad range of local clinical champions to initiate positive, transformational change and spreading good practice across the NHS. The network's core principles are to: (i) support clinical leadership engagement; (ii) improve NHS clinical service delivery; and (iii) enable clinicians to influence policy implementation by giving them direct access to local and national policy leads.

http://www.pierproject.ca/

This is the website of the PIER project, which aims to demonstrate the importance of developing trusting and supportive relationships within an interprofessional health care environment in order to encourage and sustain a strong and respectful culture. The project is funded by Health Canada and led by an interprofessional team of health care professionals from Master University Faculty of Health Sciences. Evaluation resources and methods used by the PIER project include *Practice Genograms* and the *Interdisciplinary Education Perception Scale (IEPS)*.

Index

References to Tables will be in *italics*